Toxicology of Contact Hypersensitivity

Toxicology of Contact Hypersensitivity

Edited by

IAN KIMBER

Zeneca Central Toxicology Laboratory, Alderley Park, Macclesfield, UK

and

THOMAS MAURER

Ciba-Geigy Ltd, Basel, Switzerland

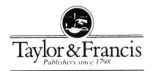

Taylor & Francis
Publishers since 1798

UK   Taylor & Francis Ltd, 1 Gunpowder Square, London EC4 3DE
USA   Taylor & Francis Inc., 1900 Frost Road, Suite 101, Bristol, PA 19007

Copyright © Taylor & Francis Ltd 1996

British Library Cataloguing in Publication Data
A catalogue record for this book is available from the British Library.
ISBN 0-7484-0349-3

Library of Congress Cataloguing Publication data are available

Cover design by Youngs Design in Production

Typeset in Times 10/12pt by Keyset Composition, Colchester, Essex
Printed in Great Britain by T. J. Press (Padstow) Ltd, Cornwall

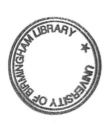

Contents

Toxicology of Contact Hypersensitivity

I. KIMBER

Zeneca Central Toxicology Laboratory, Macclesfield

T. MAURER

Ciba-Geigy Ltd, Basel

Introduction

A useful working definition of allergy is the adverse health effects which result from the stimulation of specific immune responses. Allergic disease develops normally in two temporally discrete stages. Exposure to allergen will induce in susceptible individuals the quantity and quality of immune response necessary for sensitization (the induction phase). Sensitization can be regarded simply as an acquired ability to respond immunologically to the inducing allergen in a heightened fashion. If the sensitized individual encounters the same allergen for a second or subsequent time then an accelerated and more aggressive secondary immune response will be provoked that results in the clinical features of allergic disease (the elicitation phase).

Chemicals, as well as proteins, are able to induce allergic responses and by far the most common form of allergy resulting from the exposure of predisposed individuals to small molecular weight materials is contact hypersensitivity, known also as contact or skin sensitization and allergic contact dermatitis.

Although it had been suspected previously, it was Josef Jadassohn who, at the end of the last century, confirmed that skin reactions and skin inflammation caused by certain materials could not be reconciled on the basis of irritant activity, but reflected instead some increase in sensitivity (Sulzberger, 1938). Jadassohn, in addition to making this seminal observation, was the father of patch testing which remains today the primary method available in the clinic for diagnosis of allergic contact dermatitis and for identification of the causative allergen (Jadassohn, 1896).

The pioneering work of Landsteiner and Jacobs (1935), identifying the relationship between chemical structure and immunogenicity and the subsequent studies of Landsteiner and Chase (1937, 1939, 1942) laid the foundations for future immunological investigations of the mechanistic basis for skin sensitization. The history of experimental studies designed to elucidate immunological aspects of contact sensitivity are described eloquently in a monograph published by Ladislav Polak, who himself made a remarkable contribution to the subject (Polak, 1980).

During the last quarter of a century a clearer understanding of many aspects of the immune system and its workings, including the rediscovery of epidermal Langerhans cells and their place within an integrated skin immune system, the characterization and functional diversity of T lymphocytes and the role of myriad cytokines, has yielded a more sophisticated, but as yet far from complete, appreciation of the immunobiological processes associated with the induction and expression of contact sensitization.

The phenomenon of skin sensitization attracts the interest of several scientific disciplines. To the practising dermatologist allergic contact dermatitis remains a problem and to the immunologist contact sensitization provides an endlessly fascinating model for the investigation of adaptive immune function. Contact dermatitis, including allergic contact dermatitis, resulting from exposure in the workplace to chemicals is a common occupational health problem (Mathias, 1988; Adams, 1990). As a consequence contact allergy is of considerable importance to the toxicologist who has the responsibility of identifying and characterizing the skin sensitizing potential of chemicals and estimating the risk they pose to human health.

It is the purpose of this book to draw together into a single volume experience from each of these disciplines and to illustrate the ways in which recent advances have aided the toxicologist in the identification of hazard and assessment of risk associated with skin sensitization.

References

ADAMS, R.M. (1990) *Occupational Skin Disease*, 2nd Edition, Philadelphia, Saunders.

JADASSOHN, J. (1896) Zur kenntnis der arzneiexantheme. *Archiv Dermatologische Forschung*, **34**, 103.

LANDSTEINER, K. and CHASE, M.W. (1937) Studies on the sensitization of animals with simple chemical compounds. IV. Anaphylaxis induced by picryl chloride and 2,4-dinitrochlorobenzene. *Journal of Experimental Medicine*, **66**, 337–51.

(1939) Studies on the sensitization of animals with simple chemical compounds. VI. Experiments on the sensitization of guinea pigs to poison ivy. *Journal of Experimental Medicine*, **69**, 767–85.

(1942) Experiments on transfer of cutaneous sensitivity to simple compounds. *Proceedings of the Society of Experimental Biology and Medicine*, **49**, 688–90.

LANDSTEINER, K. and JACOBS, E. (1935) Studies on the sensitization of animals with simple chemical compounds. *Journal of Experimental Medicine*, **61**, 643–66.

MATHIAS, C.G.T. (1988) Occupational dermatoses. *Journal of the American Academy of Dermatology*, **19**, 1107–14.

POLAK, L. (1980) *Immunological Aspects of Contact Sensitivity. An Experimental Study*. Monographs in Allergy Vol. 15. Basle, Karger.

SULZBERGER, M.D. (1936) Josef Jadassohn (1863–1936). *Archives of Dermatology*, **33**, 1063.

Contact Hypersensitivity: Immunological Mechanisms

I. KIMBER and R.J. DEARMAN

Zeneca Central Toxicology Laboratory, Macclesfield

Introduction

Contact allergy (allergic contact dermatitis) is a form of delayed-type hypersensitivity reaction and as such is dependent upon cell-mediated immune function and the activity of T lymphocytes. For the purposes of this chapter, the events that lead to contact sensitization of the susceptible individual, and which later result in the appearance of contact hypersensitivity reactions following subsequent exposure to the inducing allergen, can be separated into a number of stages. Following first encounter with the chemical sensitizer a pattern of changes is provoked in the skin which serves to modulate the movement and function of cutaneous dendritic cells. It is the responsibility of these cells to transport allergen in sufficient quantity and in an immunogenic form to the lymph nodes draining the site of exposure. Here responsive T lymphocytes are activated and induced to divide and differentiate. The daughter cells resulting from the proliferation of responsive lymphocytes provide immunological memory and ensure that after subsequent contact with the same chemical allergen an accelerated and more aggressive immune response will be mounted. Such secondary immune responses are stimulated in the skin and the local activation of allergen-specific T lymphocyte initiates the cutaneous inflammatory process that is recognized clinically as allergic contact dermatitis.

It is the purpose of this chapter to consider the immunobiology of contact hypersensitivity. The key cellular and molecular events will be discussed under two broad headings focusing on the induction of skin sensitization and the elicitation of contact hypersensitivity reactions.

The Induction Phase

As is described in greater detail in Chapter 3, it has been found in clinical studies of skin sensitization to 2,4-dinitrochlorobenzene (DNCB) that the local concentration of the inducing allergen is of pivotal importance in determining the extent to which sensitization will develop. Thus, it was reported that when using in all cases an identical amount of DNCB, the incidence of contact sensitization was reduced progressively as the area of skin over which the allergen was applied increased (White *et al.*, 1986). These data reveal that there exists a threshold for the development of clinically relevant levels of sensitization and suggest that local events at the site of exposure are important in ensuring that a critical amount of allergen in an immunogenic form reaches the draining lymph nodes. It is in the handling, processing, transport and presentation of allergen that cutaneous dendritic cells play an essential role.

Cutaneous Dendritic Cells

Within the epidermis there exists a contiguous network of Langerhans cells (LC). Epidermal LC form part of the wider family of dendritic cells (DC), all of which are bone marrow-derived and all of which have as their primary physiological role the processing and presentation of foreign antigen. In the epidermis LC act as sentinels of the immune system, surveying changes in the external environment and providing a 'trap' for external antigens encountered in the skin (Shelley and Juhlin, 1976). There is evidence now that, following topical exposure to contact sensitizing chemicals, LC are stimulated to leave the epidermis and to migrate, via the afferent lymphatics, to draining lymph nodes (Knight *et al.*, 1985; Macatonia *et al.*, 1986, 1987; Kinnaird *et al.*, 1989; Kimber *et al.*, 1990; Kripke *et al.*, 1990; Cumberbatch and Kimber, 1990). The cells which arrive in the lymph nodes, many of which bear high levels of antigen, localize in the paracortical (T lymphocyte) area and assume the characteristics of interdigitating DC (Cumberbatch and Kimber, 1990; Fossum, 1988). These antigen-bearing DC are potent stimulators of immune activation; they readily form stable clusters with T lymphocytes and will stimulate vigorous primary and secondary T cell proliferative responses *in vitro* (Knight *et al.*, 1985; Macatonia *et al.*, 1986; Hauser and Katz, 1988; Jones *et al.*, 1989; Gerberick *et al.*, 1990; Cumberbatch *et al.*, 1991b). Moreover, comparatively small numbers of antigen-bearing DC isolated from the draining nodes of contact sensitized mice are able effectively to transfer skin sensitization to naive syngeneic recipients (Knight *et al.*, 1985; Macatonia *et al.*, 1986; Kinnaird *et al.*, 1989; Macatonia and Knight, 1989). While it is likely that, under normal circumstances, epidermal LC represent the most important class of DC during the induction phase of contact sensitization, there is evidence for the existence of dermal dendritic cells that may also have the potential to process and present chemical allergen (Tse and Cooper, 1990; Lenz *et al.*, 1993; Nestle *et al.*, 1993; Duraiswamy *et al.*, 1994). Like LC, dermal DC express major histocompatibility class II (Ia) antigens, the membrane determinants with which foreign antigen must be associated for recognition by T lymphocytes. There is within murine epidermis, in addition to LC, a second population of DC which lack Ia antigen and express instead the Thy-1 glycoprotein and the $\gamma\delta$ T lymphocyte receptor (Bergstresser *et al.*, 1983; Tschachler *et al.*, 1983; Koning *et al.*, 1987). The view is that these Thy-1$^+$ epidermal dendritic cells do not themselves play a direct role in the presentation of antigen to T lymphocytes. They fail to migrate from the skin and do not transport allergen to draining lymph nodes (Cumberbatch and Kimber, 1990; Cumberbatch *et al.*, 1994). It can not be assumed, however, that Thy-1$^+$ DC fail to influence the process of contact sensitization. It was reported by Bigby *et al.* (1987) that the effectiveness of skin sensitization in mice is determined to some extent by the relative frequency of Thy-1$^+$ DC and LC in the epidermis at the site of exposure. Consistent with this are indications that Thy-1$^+$ DC are able to induce immunobiological tolerance (Sullivan *et al.*, 1986; Welsh and Kripke, 1990; Love-Schimenti and Kripke, 1994). In addition, it has been shown recently that, early following encounter with antigen, T lymphocytes bearing $\gamma\delta$ receptors elaborate cytokines that are known to influence the maturation of T helper (Th) cells and the characteristics of induced immune responses (Ferrick *et al.*, 1995). It will be instructive to examine whether, in response to chemical allergen, Thy-1$^+$ DC resident in the epidermis are able to respond in a similar way.

There exists an interesting functional distinction between epidermal LC and the DC into which they mature. It has been found that LC resident within the skin are relatively weak antigen presenting cells, but are able very effectively to process protein (Streilein and Grammer, 1989; Streilein *et al.*, 1990). During the period of migration from the epidermis and accumulation in draining lymph nodes antigen processing activity is lost and immuno-stimulatory potential acquired (Streilein and Grammer, 1989). The transition is of course consistent with the sentinel function of LC. In the skin their primary purpose is the recognition, internalization, processing and sub-sequent re-expression (in association with Ia determinants) of foreign antigen. It has been found that LC internalize antigen into endolysozomal compartments rich in Ia determinants (Girolomoni *et al.*, 1990; Bartosik, 1992; Reis e Sousa *et al.*, 1993; Kleijmeer *et al.*, 1994). This antigen is then transported to the draining lymph nodes where the requirement is for immunostimulatory activity and for the effective presentation of im-munogenic Ia-peptide complexes to responsive T lymphocytes. By this time processing activity, which is determined strictly by the maturational status of LC (Streilein and Grammer, 1989; Streilein *et al.*, 1990; Girolomoni *et al.*, 1990; Reis e Sousa *et al.*, 1993), has been lost.

The available evidence indicates that responsive Th cells recognize hapten, derived from the inducing chemical allergen, in association with peptides anchored to Ia antigens (Kohler *et al.*, 1995; Cavani *et al.*, 1995). In theory protein-reactive hapten might associate directly with the Ia-bound peptide. Alternatively, LC may internalize and process hapten-conjugated extracellular protein. Some metal allergens may represent a special case. Although it has been shown that nickel is recognized in association with Ia-bound peptide, it has been suggested that the recognition unit for gold-responsive T cells is the metal bound directly to the Ia molecule (Sinigaglia, 1994). The induced changes to which LC are subject and that permit the induction of contact sensitization are, to a large extent, mediated by cutaneous cytokines.

Epidermal Cytokines

The skin has been recognized for some time as an immunologically-active tissue. Cutaneous immune function is regulated by cytokines produced locally. Both keratinocytes and LC are sources of epidermal cytokines, some of which are produced constitutively, while the expression of others requires an external or paracrine stimulus. The cytokines known to be produced by epidermal cells and their cellular sources are listed in Table 2.1.

Regulation of Langerhans Cell Function

Culture of Langerhans cells in the presence of keratinocytes or keratinocyte-derived cytokines induces a functional maturation which is characterized by the acquisition of antigen presenting and immunostimulatory activity (Schuler and Steinman, 1985). The important cytokines in effecting this transition are granulocyte/macrophage colony-stimulating factor (GM-CSF), interleukin 1 (IL-1) and tumour necrosis factor α (TNF-α). The functional maturation of cultured LC is mediated primarily by GM-CSF, possibly acting in concert with IL-1 (Witmer-Pack *et al.*, 1987; Heufler *et al.*, 1988; Picut *et al.*, 1988). In contrast, TNF-α serves to maintain the viability of LC in culture without causing their maturation (Koch *et al.*, 1990). It is assumed that the changes induced in cultured LC represent an *in vitro* correlate of the immunostimulatory potential that develops as LC migrate from the skin to the lymph nodes, and that these same cytokines are important *in vivo*. Consistent with a role for these cytokines in the maturation of LC is the fact that they are each induced or upregulated following the topical exposure of mice to chemical allergens (Enk and Katz, 1992a). Moreover, low levels of GM-CSF have been found in the afferent lymph of humans exposed to the skin irritant sodium lauryl sulphate, a chemical known to cause the migration of LC in both man and mouse (Hunziker *et al.*, 1992; Brand *et al.*, 1992; Cumberbatch *et al.*, 1993).

7

Toxicology of Contact Hypersensitivity

Table 2.1 Epidermal cytokines

Cytokines	Langerhans cells	Keratinocytes
	Constitutive or inducible expression in:	
Interleukins		
Interleukin 1α (IL-1α)	−	+
Interleukin 1β (IL-1β)	+	−
Interleukin 3 (IL-3)	−	+
Interleukin 6 (IL-6)	+	+
Interleukin 7 (IL-7)	−	+
Interleukin 8 (IL-8)	−	+
Interleukin 10 (IL-10)	−	+
Interleukin 12 (IL-12)	−	+
Colony stimulating factors		
Granulocyte colony-stimulating factor (G-CSF)	−	+
Macrophage colony-stimulating factor (M-CSF)	−	+
Granulocyte/macrophage colony-stimulating factor (GM-CSF)	−	+
Transforming growth factor α (TGF-α)	−	+
Transforming growth factor β (TGF-β)	+	+
Tumour necrosis factor α (TNF-α)	−	+
Macrophage inflammatory protein 1α (MIP-1α)	+	−
Macrophage inflammatory protein 2 (MIP-2)	+	+

Summarized from available human and/or mouse studies (McKenzie and Sauder, 1990; Schreiber *et al.*, 1992; Heufler *et al.*, 1992, 1993; Gruschwitz and Hornstein, 1993; Matsue *et al.*, 1992; Enk and Katz, 1992a, b; Aragane *et al.*, 1994; Kimber 1994).

It has been shown in mice that following skin sensitization, and while in transit to the draining lymph nodes, LC are subject to a number of phenotypic changes consistent with the development of immunostimulatory activity (Kimber and Cumberbatch, 1992). Dendritic cells which arrive in the draining nodes, including antigen-bearing DC, display increased membrane Ia expression compared with epidermal LC (Cumberbatch *et al.*, 1991a). Of importance also is the fact that there is in addition a very substantial (approximately 40-fold) increase in the expression of intercellular adhesion molecule-1 (ICAM-1; CD54), a membrane determinant which has as its ligand leukocyte function antigen-1 (LFA-1) found on T lymphocytes (Cumberbatch *et al.*, 1992). Increased membrane ICAM-1 facilitates the antigen-independent association of DC with T lymphocytes as the first step

8

in the process of antigen presentation. Other receptor-ligand interactions are required for the effective activation of T lymphocytes and of particular importance in this respect are members of the B7 family. B7-1 and B7-2 act as ligands for the CTLA-4/CD28 T lymphocyte signalling system and both are expressed by DC (Larsen *et al.*, 1992; Hart *et al.*, 1993; Razi-Wolf *et al.*, 1994; Girolomoni *et al.*, 1994; Caux *et al.*, 1994; Inaba *et al.*, 1994). As both B7-1 and B7-2 are upregulated during culture of LC it can be assumed that there is a similar increased expression during LC migration *in vivo* (Larsen *et al.*, 1992; Inaba *et al.*, 1994; Girolomoni *et al.*, 1994).

In addition to effecting the maturation of LC, there is now evidence that epidermal cytokines are able to induce their movement and migration. Of particular importance is TNF-α, a product of keratinocytes that is upregulated following skin sensitization (Enk and Katz, 1992a). It has been shown that TNF-α causes the migration of LC, but not of Thy-1[+] DC, from the skin and the subsequent arrival of DC in draining lymph nodes (Cumberbatch and Kimber, 1992; Cumberbatch *et al.*, 1994). Consistent with an important role for TNF-α in the stimulation of LC migration is the fact that systemic treatment of mice with a neutralizing anti-TNF-α antibody serves to inhibit the accumulation of DC in draining nodes normally associated with skin sensitization (Cumberbatch and Kimber, 1995). The induction of TNF-α may itself be regulated in paracrine fashion. It has been demonstrated that the optimal induction of contact sensitization in mice is dependent upon the availability of interleukin 1β (IL-1β) (Enk *et al.*, 1993a), a cytokine product of LC that is upregulated very rapidly following topical application of chemical allergens (Enk and Katz, 1992a). This cytokine is known to influence the expression of other epidermal cytokines and of cytokine receptors and will stimulate a substantial upregulation of TNF-α and of TNF-α and GM-CSF receptors (Winzen *et al.*, 1993; Enk *et al.*, 1993a; Kampgen *et al.*, 1994). The following sequence of events suggests itself. As an early event following skin sensitization LC are stimulated, possibly via the direct interaction of the chemical with membrane Ia (Trede *et al.*, 1991), to produce IL-1β. This cytokine acts in paracrine fashion to stimulate the increased production by keratinocytes of TNF-α, and may serve also to induce in an autocrine manner the increased expression by LC of receptors for both TNF-α and GM-CSF. Keratinocyte-derived TNF-α will then act on LC, via the 75 kDa (TNF-R2) receptor for TNF-α, to trigger migration from the skin.

It is worth considering what effects TNF-α and other cytokines may exert on LC and the surrounding tissue matrix to facilitate migration. Both LC and keratinocytes express the homotypic adhesion molecule E-cadherin. It has been proposed that it is this molecule that retains LC within the epidermis; the implication being that a prerequisite for migration is the reduced expression of E-cadherin by one or other cell type (Tang *et al.*, 1993; Blauvelt *et al.*, 1995). Certainly it is the case that, compared with LC in the epidermis, the DC found within lymph nodes express significantly less

E-cadherin (Borkowski *et al.*, 1994). Other adhesion molecules may also play important roles in the movement of LC. As described previously, the functional maturation of LC is associated with a very substantial increase in expression of ICAM-1. It now appears that this molecule may be relevant not only for interaction with T lymphocytes, but also for LC traffic. Recent investigations have revealed that treatment of mice with a combination of anti-ICAM-1 and anti-LFA-1 monoclonal antibodies inhibited completely the arrival of antigen-bearing DC in draining lymph nodes and the induction of skin sensitization (Ma *et al.*, 1994).

The sum effect of the cascade of events induced in the skin and that results in the accumulation of antigen-bearing dendritic cells in the draining lymph nodes provides for the central event in contact sensitization, the stimulation of appropriate T lymphocyte responses. A question posed frequently is why chemicals cause contact sensitization, or rather what properties must a chemical possess to induce allergic responses. One view is that a better way of formulating this question is to ask what serves to prevent chemicals encountered on the skin from provoking sensitization; all chemicals, in theory, being exogenous antigens. The successful stimulation of skin sensitization in fact requires that a number of important biological criteria be fulfilled. The chemical must have the physiochemical characteristics to permit absorption across the stratum corneum. Potentially strong chemical allergens which are unable to gain access to the viable epidermis will fail to stimulate a cutaneous immune response. While chemicals represent antigenic epitopes these are haptens which must associate with protein to generate an immunogenic moiety. Some degree of protein reactivity is therefore necessary. Finally, as described above, a complex series of events must be induced in the skin to allow the migration and functional activation of Langerhans cells and/or other cutaneous dendritic cells. These events are initiated and regulated by epidermal cytokines and exposure to chemical must result in a sufficiently strong signal to provoke local cytokine production. It has long been considered that some limited irritation at the site of exposure to contact allergens facilitates the development of skin sensitization. It may be that some degree of skin trauma is required for the efficient upregulation of relevant epidermal cytokines. If a chemical is inherently antigenic, is able to induce epidermal cytokine production and gain access through the stratum corneum and is able also to associate in some form with cellular or extracellular protein, then sensitization may be induced. If all the criteria are met then a T lymphocyte response will be stimulated.

T Lymphocyte Responses

It is assumed usually that contact sensitization and the elicitation of dermal hypersensitivity reactions depend primarily upon CD4$^+$ Th cells. However, allergen-specific CD8$^+$ cells are induced also (Fehr *et al.*, 1994) and may play a role (Gocinski and Tigelaar, 1990). The extent and duration of T lymphocyte activation in the draining nodes, as measured by cellular proliferation, is an important determinant of contact sensitization (Kimber and Dearman, 1991). T lymphocyte proliferative activity induced following topical exposure to chemical allergens is subject to homeostatic control mechanisms which regulate the extent to which sensitization develops (Kimber *et al.*, 1989, 1991; Baker *et al.*, 1991).

In addition to quantitative aspects of T lymphocyte activation, the quality of immune response provoked is of pivotal importance. It is now accepted that there exists in both man and mouse a functional heterogeneity among CD4$^+$ Th cells. Two main populations are recognized and have been designated Th1 and Th2 (Mosmann *et al.*, 1986, 1991; Mosmann and Coffman, 1989; Romagnani, 1991; Romagnani *et al.*, 1992). The major functional distinction between these subsets resides in their cytokine secretion profiles. Both populations produce GM-CSF and interleukin 3 (IL-3). However, only Th1 cells elaborate interleukin 2 (IL-2), interferon γ (IFN-γ) and tumour necrosis factor β (TNF-β; lymphotoxin) and only Th2 cells produce interleukins 4, 5, 6 and 10 (IL-4, IL-5, IL-6 and IL-10) (Mosmann and Coffman, 1989; Mosmann *et al.*, 1991). These populations can be regarded as the most differentiated forms of CD4$^+$ cells and develop from a common precursor as the immune response matures (Mosmann *et al.*, 1991; Bendelac and Schwartz, 1991). The characteristics of activated CD4$^+$ T lymphocytes, and the balance between Th1 and Th2 cells, have a profound influence on the nature of induced immune responses. The selective stimulation of Th2 cells favours the development of humoral immune responses and is necessary for the induction and maintenance of IgE antibody production (Finkelman *et al.*, 1988; Mosmann *et al*, 1991). In contrast, Th1 cells effect delayed-type hypersensitivity reactions and their cytokine product IFN-γ plays an important role in this process (Cher and Mosmann, 1987; Fong and Mosmann, 1989; Diamanstein *et al.*, 1988). It is assumed therefore that the effectiveness of skin sensitization and the vigour of contact hypersensitivity reactions will be determined to an important extent by the availability of allergen-reactive Th1 cells. In this context it has been found in mice that contact allergens stimulate preferential Th1-type immune responses, whereas chemicals known to cause respiratory sensitization and to provoke IgE antibody production induce instead selective Th2 cell activation (Dearman and Kimber, 1991, 1992; Dearman *et al.*, 1992a, b, c, 1994). In humans also contact hypersensitivity is associated usually with Th1-type cells. The majority of T cell clones generated from the peripheral blood of nickel-sensitive donors has been shown to produce high levels of IFN-γ, but only low or undetectable levels of the Th2 cell cytokines IL-4 and IL-5 (Kapsenberg *et al.*, 1991, 1992). In contrast, atopic dermatitis, allergic asthma and other IgE-mediated hypersensitivity reactions are in man characterized by the presence of Th2-type cells (Kay *et al.*, 1991; van der Heijden *et al.*, 1991; Durham *et al.*, 1992; Robinson *et al.*, 1992, 1993).

The signals and immunoregulatory mechanisms that result in the selective development of Th cell subpopulations while not clearly understood are likely to involve the characteristics of the inducing antigen itself, the extent, duration and route of exposure and the characteristics of antigen processing and presenting cells (Weaver *et al.*, 1988; Chang *et al.*, 1990; Gajewski *et al.*, 1991; Saito *et al.*, 1994). Of particular relevance potentially is heat-stable antigen (HSA), a costimulatory molecule for CD4$^+$ T lymphocytes expressed on LC and that may be required for the antigen-driven activation of Th1 cells (Enk and Katz, 1994).

Probably the most important determinant of selective Th cell maturation is the relative availability in the local microenvironment of cytokines themselves (Swain *et al.*, 1991; Coffman *et al.*, 1991; Abehsira-Amar *et al.*, 1992; Hsieh *et al.*, 1992). Cytokines of Th1-type favour the development of Th1 cell responses while IL-4, IL-10 and other Th2 cytokines favour preferential Th2 cell responses. Moreover, these cytokines have mutually antagonistic effects so, however first induced, preferential Th cell subset responses will be maintained and amplified by their own cytokine products. Of particular importance for regulation of the induction and elicitation of contact allergy appears to be IL-10, a cytokine described originally as cytokine synthesis inhibitory factor. It has been found recently that IL-10, a product of keratinocytes as well as of Th2 cells, will inhibit the immunostimulatory and antigen presenting functions of LC and the ability of dendritic cells to induce IFN-γ production by T lymphocytes (Enk *et al.*, 1993b; Macatonia *et al.*, 1993; Peguet-Navarro *et al.*, 1994; Beissert *et al.*, 1995). Moreover IL-10 inhibits the elicitation of contact and delayed-hypersensitivity reactions in previously sensitized mice (Li *et al.*, 1994; Kondo *et al.*, 1994).

The source of the cytokines that initially drive CD4$^+$ T lymphocytes toward a phenotype of selective cytokine expression may lie outside the classical adaptive immune system with natural killer (NK) cells, mast cells and T cells bearing the γδ receptor all having important, but different, roles (Romagnani, 1992; Ferrick *et al.*, 1995). With respect to the selective development of Th1 cells, the production of interleukin 12 (IL-12), previously designated natural killer cell stimulatory factor, may represent a pivotal first step in the maturation process. This molecule is secreted by a variety of cell types, inducing B lymphocytes and macrophages, and stimulates NK cells and T lymphocytes to produce IFN-γ (Chan *et al.*, 1991). Importantly, IL-12 promotes the differentiation of IFN-γ secreting T lymphocytes and inhibits the development of Th2-type (IL-4 producing) cells (Manetti *et al.*, 1993; Trinchieri, 1994). The role of IL-12 in CD4$^+$ Th1 cell development is complicated insofar as it appears to have a dual role. IL-12 stimulates the production of IFN-γ by NK cells and other populations and also acts together with IFN-γ in driving Th1 cell maturation directly (Schmitt *et al.*, 1994). Perhaps not unexpectedly, therefore, Maguire (1995) has demonstrated that local injection of recombinant IL-12 will enhance the induction of skin

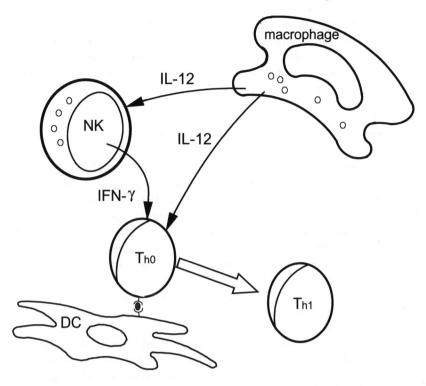

Figure 2.1 The role of cytokines in the development of Th1-type immune responses

sensitization in mice. Some of the factors that promote the development and function of Th1 cells are illustrated in Figure 2.1.

In summary, the weight of evidence indicates that during the induction phase of skin sensitization there is a selective drive toward the development of allergen-specific Th1 cells and that these populations are primarily responsible for the subsequent elicitation of challenge-induced cutaneous hypersensitivity reactions. It is possible, however, that the situation may be more complicated than the above analysis implies. Two other factors have to be taken into consideration, the first of which is that there is now growing evidence for a similar, although not necessarily identical, functional heterogeneity among CD8$^+$ T lymphocytes (Le Gros and Erard, 1994; Kemeny *et al.*, 1994; Croft *et al.*, 1994). It is possible that CD8$^+$ cells may, via cytokine production, influence the development and/or maintenance of differentiated CD4$^+$ populations, or may serve directly to influence the induction and elicitation of contact hypersensitivity. The second issue regards the role of IL-4 and IL-4-producing cells in the expression of contact hypersensitivity reactions. It has been suggested recently that in humans mRNA for IL-4 is expressed strongly in allergic contact dermatitis skin lesions (Ohmen *et al.*, 1995). Associated with this are the results of a recent experimental study in which it was found that treatment of mice with a neutralizing anti-IL-4 antibody inhibited the elicitation of contact hypersensitivity (Salerno *et al.*, 1995). These observations suggest that the optimal elicitation of allergic contact hypersensitivity may require IL-4 in addition to Th1 effector cells.

The Elicitation Phase

The expanded populations of allergen-reactive T lymphocytes which result from the stimulation of an immune response following first encounter with the chemical sensitizer distribute systemically. Following subsequent topical exposure to the same chemical these T lymphocytes will recognize and respond to allergen in the skin and initiate a local inflammatory response.

The whole process of T cell-mediated immune effector function in the skin is dependent upon the arrival and accumulation of allergen-responsive memory cells at the site of challenge. This is facilitated by mechanisms that permit the selective recruitment of memory, rather than naive, T lymphocytes to the skin and that encourage the return to the skin of T cells reactive with antigens first encountered there.

Naive and memory/effector T lymphocytes may be distinguished as a function of CD45 (common leukocyte) antigen expression. Virgin T lymphocytes that have not yet responded to antigens with which they are reactive express the high molecular weight isoform of CD45, designated CD45RA. Memory/effector T cells express, in contrast, a truncated form of the molecule, CD45RO (Akbar *et al.*, 1988). It has been found in contact hypersensitivity reactions, and at the sites of other forms of skin lesion, that it is CD45RO$^+$ T cells which predominate (Silvennoinen-Kassinen *et al.*, 1992; Markey *et al.*, 1990; Frew and Kay, 1991). The vast majority of skin-infiltrating memory T lymphocytes express also the oligosaccharide determinant cutaneous lymphocyte-associated antigen (CLA), a molecule that is closely related to sialyl Lewis X. Only a small proportion of T cells found in the peripheral blood or in extracutaneous tissue express this molecule (Picker *et al.*, 1990, 1993). The transmigration of skin-homing memory T cells is effected by interaction between CLA and E-selectin, one of several adhesion molecules that may be induced or upregulated by cytokines on vascular endothelium (Picker *et al.*, 1991; Griffiths *et al.*, 1991; Bevilacqua, 1993). Transendothelial migration of lymphocytes into skin may involve also interactions with other inducible endothelial adhesion molecules such as vascular cell adhesion molecule-1 (VCAM-1) and ICAM-1 by determinants (VLA-4 [very late antigen-4] and LFA-1, respectively) expressed by T lymphocytes (Silber *et al.*, 1994; Santamaria Babi *et al.*, 1995). Following the selective recruitment of T cells from the circulation further progress into skin sites will depend upon interaction with the tissue matrix and movement along chemotactic gradients. Important for the accumulation

14

of cells at reactive sites is interleukin 8, a product of keratinocytes and a strong T lymphocyte chemoattractant (Griffiths *et al.*, 1991; Barker *et al.*, 1991). Once infiltrating T cells have responded to antigen then their production of IFN-γ will serve to encourage further the recruitment of lymphocytes to inflammatory sites (Issekutz *et al.*, 1988).

Memory $CD4^+$ T lymphocytes will recognize and respond to antigen in the context of membrane Ia. It is well established that requirements for the antigen-driven activation of memory cells are less rigorous than those necessary for the initial stimulation of naive lymphocytes. For activation of unprimed T lymphocytes mature dendritic cells are necessary for effective antigen presentation. In contrast, other Ia^+ populations, including resident epidermal LC, may stimulate secondary responses by T lymphocytes. In inflamed skin the expression by keratinocytes of Ia and ICAM-1 is induced by TNF-α and IFN-γ (Basham *et al.*, 1984; Dustin *et al.*, 1988; Griffiths *et al.*, 1989). It is possible that Ia^+ keratinocytes will present antigen to responsive $CD4^+$ memory T lymphocytes.

The elicitation phase of contact hypersensitivity is therefore characterized by the selective recruitment of allergen-reactive skin-homing memory T lymphocytes, their subsequent activation and associated cytokine production, which in turn results in further leukocyte infiltration and the development of a cutaneous inflammatory reaction. As described previously the expression of challenge-induced contact hypersensitivity reactions is subject to regulatory controls, notably those mediated by IL-10 which serves to inhibit IFN-γ expression and also reduces induced increases in vasopermeability (Kondo *et al.*, 1994; Li *et al.*, 1994). Like the induction phase of sensitization, the elicitation, duration and severity of contact hypersensitivity is to a large extent regulated by the action of cytokines.

References

ABEHSIRA-AMAR, O., GILBERT, M., JOLIY, M., THEZE, J. and JANKOVIC, D.L., 1992, IL-4 plays a dominant role in the differential development of Th_0 into Th_1, and Th_2 cells, *Journal of Immunology*, **148**, 3820–9.

AKBAR, A.N., TERRY, L., TIMMS, A., BEVERLEY, P.C.L. and JANOSSY, G., 1988, Loss of CD45R and gain of UCHL1 reactivity is a feature of primed T cells, *Journal of Immunology*, **140**, 2171–8.

ARAGANE, Y., REIMANN, H., BHARDWAJ, R.S., SCHWARTZ, A., SAWADA, Y., YAMADA, H., LUGER, T.A., KUBIN, M., TRINCHIERI, G. and SCHWARTZ, T., 1994, IL-12 is expressed and released by human keratinocytes and epidermoid carcinoma cell lines, *Journal of Immunology*, **153**, 5366–72.

BAKER, D., KIMBER, I., AHMED, K. and TURK, J.L., 1991, Antigen-specific and non-specific depression of proliferative responses during induced contact sensitivity in mice, *International Journal of Experimental Pathology*, **72**, 55–65.

BARKER, J.N.W.N., JONES, M.L., MITRA, R.S., FANTONE, J.C., KUNKEL, S.L., DIXIT, V.M. and NICKOLOFF, B.J., 1991, Modulation of keratinocyte-derived interleukin-8 which is chemotactic for neutrophils and T lymphocytes, *American*

Journal of Pathology, **139**, 869–76.

BARTOSIK, J., 1992, Cytomembrane-derived Birbeck granules transport horseradish peroxidase to the endosomal compartment in the human Langerhans cell, *Journal of Investigative Dermatology*, **99**, 53–8.

BASHAM, T.Y., NICKOLOFF, B.J., MERIGAN, T.C. and MORHENN, V.B., 1984, Recombinant gamma interferon induces HLA-DR on cultured human keratinocytes, *Journal of Investigative Dermatology*, **83**, 88–92.

BEISSERT, S., HOSOI, J., GRABBE, S., ASAHINA, A. and GRANSTEIN, R.D., 1995, IL-10 inhibits tumor antigen presentation by epidermal antigen-presenting cells, *Journal of Immunology*, **154**, 1280–6.

BENDELAC, A. and SCHWARTZ, R.H., 1991, Tho cells in the thymus. The question of T-helper lineages, *Immunological Reviews*, **123**, 169–88.

BERGSTRESSER, P.R., TIGELAAR, R.E., DEES, J.H. and STREILEIN, J.W., 1983, Thy-1 antigen-bearing dendritic cells populate murine epidermis, *Journal of Investigative Dermatology*, **81**, 286–8.

BEVILACQUA, M.P., 1993, Endothelial-leukocyte adhesion molecules, *Annual Review of Immunology*, **11**, 767–804.

BIGBY, M., KWAN, T. and SY, M-S., 1987, Ratio of Langerhans cells to Thy-1[+] dendritic epidermal cells influences the intensity of contact hypersensitivity, *Journal of Investigative Dermatology*, **89**, 495–9.

BLAUVELT, A., KATZ, S.I. and UDEY, M.C., 1995, Human Langerhans cells express E-cadherin, *Journal of Investigative Dermatology*, **104**, 293–6.

BORKOWSKI, T.A., VAN DYKE, B.J., SCHWARZENBERGER, K., McFARLAND, V.W., FARR, A.G. and UDEY, M.C., 1994, Expression of E-cadherin by murine dendritic cells : E-cadherin as a dendritic cell differentiation antigen characteristic of epidermal Langerhans cells and related cells, *European Journal of Immunology*, **24**, 2767–74.

BRAND, C.U., HUNZIKER, T. and BRAATHEN, L.R., 1992, Isolation of human skin-derived lymph: flow and output of cells following sodium lauryl sulphate-induced contact dermatitis, *Archives of Dermatological Research*, **284**, 123–8.

CAUX, C., VANBERVLIET, B., MASSACRIER, C., AZUMA, M., OKUMURA, K., LANIER, L.L. and BANCHEREAU, J. 1994, B70/B7-2 is identical to CD86 and is the major functional ligand for CD28 expressed on human dendritic cells, *Journal of Experimental Medicine*, **180**, 1841–7.

CAVANI, A., HACKETT, C.J., WILSON, K.J., ROTHBARD, J.B. and KATZ, S.I., 1995, Characterization of epitopes recognized by hapten-specific CD4[+] T cells, *Journal of Immunology*, **154**, 1232–8.

CHAN, S.H., PERUSSIA, B., GUPTA, J.W., KOBAYASHI, M., POSPISIL, M., YOUNG, H.A., WOLF, S.F., YOUNG, D., CLARK, S.C. and TRINCHIERI, G., 1991, Induction of interferon γ production by natural killer cell stimulatory factor: characterization of the responder cells and synergy with other inducers, *Journal of Experimental Medicine*, **173**, 869–79.

CHANG, T-L., SHEA, C.M., URIOSTE, S., THOMPSON, R.C., BOOM, W.H. and ABBAS, A.K., 1990, Heterogeneity of helper/inducer T lymphocytes. III. Responses of IL-2- and IL-4-producing (Th1 and Th2) clones to antigens presented by different accessory cells, *Journal of Immunology*, **145**, 2803–8.

CHER, D.J. and MOSMANN, T.R., 1987, Two types of murine helper T cell clones. II. Delayed type hypersensitivity is mediated by Th1 clones, *Journal of Immunology*, **138**, 3688–94.

COFFMAN, R.L., VARKILA, K., SCOTT, P. and CHATELAIN, R., 1991, Role of cytokines in the differentiation of CD4$^+$ T-cell subsets in vivo, *Immunological Reviews*, **123**, 189–207.

CROFT, M., CARTER, L., SWAIN, S.L. and DUTTON, R.W., 1994, Generation of polarized antigen-specific CD8 effector populations: reciprocal action of interleukin (IL)-4 and IL-12 in promoting type 2 versus type 1 cytokine profiles, *Journal of Experimental Medicine*, **180**, 1715–28.

CUMBERBATCH, M. and KIMBER, I., 1990, Phenotypic characteristics of antigen-bearing cells in the draining lymph nodes of contact-sensitized mice, *Immunology*, **71**, 404–10.

1992, Dermal tumour necrosis factor-α induces dendritic cell migration to draining lymph nodes, and possibly provides one stimulus for Langerhans cell migration, *Immunology*, **75**, 257–63.

1995, Tumour necrosis factor-α is required for accumulation of dendritic cells in draining lymph nodes and for optimal contact sensitization, *Immunology*, **84**, 31–5.

CUMBERBATCH, M., FIELDING, I. and KIMBER, I., 1994, Modulation of epidermal Langerhans cell frequency by tumour necrosis factor-α, *Immunology*, **81**, 395–401.

CUMBERBATCH, M., GOULD, S.J., PETERS, S.W. and KIMBER, I., 1991a, MHC class II expression by Langerhans cells and lymph node dendritic cells: possible evidence for the maturation of Langerhans cells following contact sensitization, *Immunology*, **74**, 414–9.

CUMBERBATCH, M., ILLINGWORTH, I. and KIMBER, I., 1991b, Antigen-bearing dendritic cells in the draining lymph nodes of contact sensitized mice: cluster formation with lymphocytes, *Immunology*, **74**, 139–45.

CUMBERBATCH, M., PETERS, S.W., GOULD, S.J. and KIMBER, I., 1992, Intercellular adhesion molecule-1 (ICAM-1) expression by lymph node dendritic cells: comparison with epidermal Langerhans cells, *Immunology Letters*, **32**, 105–10.

CUMBERBATCH, M., SCOTT, R.C., BASKETTER, D.A., SCHOLES, E.W., HILTON, J., DEARMAN, R.J. and KIMBER, I., 1993, Influence of sodium lauryl sulphate on 2,4-dinitrochlorobenzene-induced lymph node activation, *Toxicology*, **77**, 181–91.

DEARMAN, R.J. and KIMBER, I., 1991, Differential stimulation of immune function by respiratory and contact chemical allergens, *Immunology*, **72**, 563–70.

1992, Divergent immune responses to respiratory and contact chemical allergens: antibody elicited by phthalic anhydride and oxazolone, *Clinical and Experimental Allergy*, **22**, 241–50.

DEARMAN, R.J., BASKETTER, D.A., COLEMAN, J.W. and KIMBER, I., 1992a, The cellular and molecular basis for divergent allergic responses to chemicals, *Chemical-Biological Interactions*, **84**, 1–10.

DEARMAN, R.J., MITCHELL, J.A., BASKETTER, D.A. and KIMBER, I., 1992b, Differential ability of occupational chemical contact and respiratory allergens to cause immediate and delayed dermal hypersensitivity reactions in mice, *International Archives of Allergy and Immunology*, **97**, 315–21.

DEARMAN, R.J., RAMDIN, L.S.P., BASKETTER, D.A. and KIMBER, I., 1994, Inducible interleukin-4-secreting cells provoked in mice during chemical sensitization, *Immunology*, **81**, 551–7.

17

DEARMAN, R.J., SPENCE, L.M. and KIMBER, I., 1992c, Characterization of murine immune responses to allergenic diisocyanates, *Toxicology and Applied Pharmacology*, **112**, 190–7.

DIAMANSTEIN, T., ECKERT, R., VOLK, H-D. and KUPIER-WEGLINSKI, J-W., 1988, Reversal by interferon-γ of inhibition of delayed-type hypersensitivity induction by anti-CD4 or anti-interleukin 2 receptor (CD25) monoclonal antibodies. Evidence for the physiological role of the $CD4^+$ $Th1^+$ subset in mice, *European Journal of Immunology*, **181**, 2101–3.

DURAISWAMY, N., TSE, Y., HAMMERBERG, C., KANG, S. and COOPER, K.D., 1994, Distinction of class II MHC^+ Langerhans cell-like interstitial antigen-presenting cells in murine dermis from dermal macrophages, *Journal of Investigative Dermatology*, **103**, 678–83.

DURHAM, S.R., YING, S., VARNEY, V.A., JACOBSON, M.R., SUDDERICK, R.M., MACKAY, I.S., KAY, A.B. and HAMID, Q.A., 1992, Cytokine messenger RNA expression for IL-3, IL-4, IL-5 and granulocyte/macrophage colony-stimulating factor in the nasal mucosa after local allergen provocation: relationship to tissue eosinophilia, *Journal of Immunology*, **148**, 2390–4.

DUSTIN, M.L., SINGER, K.H., TUCK, D.T. and SPRINGER, T.A., 1988, Adhesion of T lymphocytes to epithelial keratinocytes is regulated by interferon-gamma and is mediated by intercellular adhesion molecule-1 (ICAM-1), *Journal of Experimental Medicine*, **167**, 1323–40.

ENK, A.H., ANGELONI, V.L., UDEY, M.C. and KATZ, S.I., 1993a, An essential role for Langerhans cell-derived IL-1β in the initiation of primary immune responses in skin, *Journal of Immunology*, **150**, 3698–704.

1993b, Inhibition of Langerhans cell antigen-presenting function by IL-10. A role for IL-10 in induction of tolerance, *Journal of Immunology*, **151**, 2390–8.

ENK, A.H. and KATZ, S.I., 1992a, Early molecular events in the induction phase of contact sensitivity, *Proceedings of the National Academy of Sciences, USA*, **89**, 1398–402.

1992b, Identification and induction of keratinocyte-derived IL-10, *Journal of Immunology*, **149**, 92–5.

1994, Heat-stable antigen is an important costimulatory molecule on epidermal Langerhans cells, *Journal of Immunology*, **152**, 3264–70.

FEHR, B.S., TAKASHIMA, A., MATSUE, H., GEROMETTA, J.S., BERGSTRESSER, P.R. and CRUZ, P.D. Jr., 1994, Contact sensitization induces proliferation of heterogenous populations of hapten-specific T cells, *Experimental Dermatology*, **3**, 189–97.

FERRICK, D.A., SCHRENZEL, M.D., MULVANIA, T., HSIEH, B., FERLIN, W.G. and LEPPER, H., 1995, Differential production of interferon-γ and interleukin-4 in response to Th1- and Th2-stimulatory pathogens by $\gamma\delta$ T cells in vivo, *Nature*, **373**, 255–7.

FINKELMAN, F.D., KATONA, I.M., URBAN, J.F. Jr., HOLMES, J., OHARA, J., TUNG, A.S., SAMPLE, J.G. and PAUL, W.E., 1988, IL-4 is required to generate and sustain in vivo IgE responses, *Journal of Immunology*, **141**, 2335–41.

FONG, T.A.T. and MOSMANN, T.R., 1989, The role of IFN-γ in delayed-type hypersensitivity mediated by Th1 clones, *Journal of Immunology*, **143**, 2887–93.

FOSSUM, S., 1988, Lymph-borne dendritic leukocytes do not recirculate, but enter the lymph node paracortex to become interdigitating cells, *Scandinavian Journal of Immunology*, **27**, 97–105.

FREW, A.J. and KAY, A.B., 1991, UCHL1$^+$ (CD45RO$^+$) 'memory' T-cells predominate in the CD4$^+$ cellular infiltrate associated with allergen-induced late-phase skin reactions in atopic subjects, *Clinical and Experimental Immunology*, **84**, 270–4.

GAJEWSKI, T.F., PINNAS, M., WONG, T. and FITCH, F.W., 1991, Murine Th1 and Th2 clones proliferate optimally in response to distinct antigen-presenting cell populations, *Journal of Immunology*, **146**, 1750–8.

GERBERICK, G.F., RYAN, C.A., FLETCHER, E.R., SNELLER, D.L. and ROBINSON, M.K., 1990, An optimized lymphocyte blastogenesis assay for detecting the response of contact sensitized or photosensitized lymphocytes to hapten or photohapten modified antigen presenting cells, *Toxicology in Vitro*, **4**, 289–92.

GIROLOMONI, G., CRUZ, P.D. Jr. and BERGSTRESSER, P.R., 1990, Internalization and acidification of surface HLA-DR molecules by epidermal Langerhans cells: a paradigm for antigen processing, *Journal of Investigative Dermatology*, **94**, 753–60.

GIROLOMONI, G., ZAMBRUNO, G., MANFREDINI, R., ZACCHI, V., FERRARI, S., COSSARIZZA, A. and GIANETTI, A., 1994, Expression of B7 costimulatory molecule in cultured human epidermal Langerhans cells is regulated at the mRNA level, *Journal of Investigative Dermatology*, **103**, 54–9.

GOCINSKI, B.L. and TIGELAAR, R.E., 1990, Roles of CD4$^+$ and CD8$^+$ T cells in murine contact sensitivity revealed by in vivo monoclonal antibody depletion, *Journal of Immunology*, **144**, 4121–8.

GRIFFITHS, C.E.M., BARKER, J.N.W.N., KUNKEL, S. and NICKOLOFF, B.J., 1991, Modulation of leukocyte adhesion molecules, a T-cell chemotaxin (IL-8) and a regulatory cytokine (TNF-alpha) in allergic contact dermatitis (rhus dermatitis), *British Journal of Dermatology*, **14**, 519–26.

GRIFFITHS, C.E.M., VORHEES, J.J. and NICKOLOFF, B.J., 1989, Characterization of intercellular adhesion molecule-1 and HLA-DR in normal and inflamed skin: modulation by interferon-gamma and tumour necrosis factor, *Journal of American Academy of Dermatology*, **20**, 617–29.

GRUSCHWITZ, M.S. and HORNSTEIN, O.P., 1992, Expression of transforming growth factor type beta on human epidermal dendritic cells, *Journal of Investigative Dermatology*, **99**, 114–6.

HART, D.N.J., STARLING, G.C., CALDER, V.L. and FERNANDO, N.S., 1993, B7/BB-1 is a leukocyte differentiation antigen on human dendritic cells induced by activation, *Immunology*, **79**, 616–20.

HAUSER, C. and KATZ, S.I., 1988, Activation and expansion of hapten- and protein-specific T helper cells from non-sensitized mice, *Proceedings of the National Academy of Sciences, USA*, **85**, 5625–8.

HEUFLER, C., KOCH, F. and SCHULER, G., 1988, Granulocyte/macrophage colony-stimulating factor and interleukin 1 mediate the maturation of murine epidermal Langerhans cells into potent immunostimulatory dendritic cells, *Journal of Experimental Medicine*, **167**, 700–5.

HEUFLER, C., TOPAR, G., GRASSEGER, A., STANZL, U., KOCH, F., ROMANI, N., NAMEN, A.E. and SCHULER, G., 1993, Interleukin 7 is produced by murine and human keratinocytes, *Journal of Experimental Medicine*, **178**, 1109–14.

HEUFLER, C., TOPAR, G., KOCH, F., TROCKENBACHER, B., KAMPGEN, E., ROMANI, N. and SCHULER, G. 1992, Cytokine gene expression in murine epidermal cell suspensions: interleukin 1β and macrophage inflammatory protein 1α are selectively expresssed in Langerhans cells but are differentially regulated in culture, *Journal of Experimental Medicine*, **176**, 1221–6.

HSIEH, C-S., HEIMBERGER, A.B., GOLD, J.S., O'GARRA, A. and MURPHY, K.M., 1992, Differential regulation of T helper phenotype development by interleukins 4 and 10 in an $\alpha\beta$ T-cell-receptor transgenic system, *Proceedings of the National Academy of Sciences, USA*, **89**, 6065–9.

HUNZIKER, T., BRAND, C.U., KAPP, A., WAELTI, E.R. and BRAATHEN, L.R., 1992, Increased levels of inflammatory cytokines in human skin lymph derived from sodium lauryl sulphate-induced contact dermatitis, *British Journal of Dermatology*, **127**, 254–7.

INABA, K., WITMER-PACK, M., INABA, M., HATHCOCK, K.S., SAKUTA, H., AZUMA, M., YAGITA, H., OKUMURA, K., LINSLEY, P.S., IKEHARA, S., MURAMATSU, S., HODES, R.J. and STEINMAN, R.M., 1994, The tissue distribution of the B7-2 costimulator in mice: abundant expression on dendritic cells in situ and during maturation in vitro, *Journal of Experimental Medicine*, **180**, 1849–60.

ISSEKUTZ, T.B., STOLTZ, J.M. and MEIDE, P., 1988, Lymphocyte recruitment in delayed-type hypersensitivity. The role of IFN-γ, *Journal of Immunology*, **140**, 2989–93.

JONES, D.A., MORRIS, A.G. and KIMBER, I., 1989, Assessment of the functional activity of antigen-bearing dendritic cells isolated from the lymph nodes of contact-sensitized mice, *International Archives of Allergy and Applied Immunology*, **90**, 230–6.

KAMPGEN, E., KOCH, F., HEUFLER, C., EGGERT, A., GILL, L., GILLIS, S., DOWER, S., ROMANI, N. and SCHULER, G., 1994, Understanding the dendritic cell lineage through study of cytokine receptors, *Journal of Experimental Medicine*, **179**, 1767–76.

KAPSENBERG, M.L., WIERENGA, E.A., BOS, J.D. and JANSEN, H.M., 1991, Functional subsets of allergen-reactive human CD4$^+$ T cells, *Immunology Today*, **12**, 392–5.

KAPSENBERG, M.L., WIERENGA, E.A., STIEKMA, F.E.M., TIGGELMAN, A.M.B.C. and BOS, J.D., 1992, T$_{H1}$ lymphokine production profiles of nickel-specific CD4$^+$ T lymphocyte clones from nickel contact allergic and non-allergic individuals, *Journal of Investigative Dermatology*, **98**, 59–63.

KAY, A.B., YING, S., VARNEY, V., GAGA, M., DURHAM, S.R., MOQBEL, R., WARDLAW, A.J. and HAMID, Q., 1991, Messenger RNA expression of the cytokine gene cluster, interleukin 3 (IL-3), IL-4, IL-5 and granulocyte/macrophage colony-stimulating factor, in allergen-induced late-phase cutaneous reactions in atopic subjects, *Journal of Experimental Medicine*, **173**, 775–8.

KEMENY, D.M., NOBLE, A., HOLMES, B.J. and DIAZ-SANCHEZ, D., 1994, Immune regulation : a new role for the CD8$^+$ T cell, *Immunology Today*, **15**, 107–10.

KIMBER, I., 1994, Cytokines and the regulation of allergic sensitization to chemicals, *Toxicology*, **93**, 1–11.

KIMBER, I. and CUMBERBATCH, M., 1992, Dendritic cells and cutaneous immune responses to chemical allergens, *Toxicology and Applied Pharmacology*, **117**, 137–46.

KIMBER, I. and DEARMAN, R.J., 1991, Investigation of lymph node cell proliferation as a possible immunological correlate of contact sensitizing potential, *Food and Chemical Toxicology*, **29**, 125–9.

KIMBER, I., FOSTER, J.R., BAKER, D. and TURK, J.L., 1991, Selective impairment of T lymphocyte activation following contact sensitization with oxazolone, *International Archives of Allergy and Applied Immunology*, **95**, 142–8.

KIMBER, I., KINNAIRD, A., PETERS, S.W., and MITCHELL, J.A., 1990, Correlation between lymphocyte proliferative responses and dendritic cell migration to regional lymph nodes following skin painting with contact-sensitizing agents, *International Archives of Allergy and Applied Immunology*, **93**, 47–53.

KIMBER, I., SHEPHERD, C.J., MITCHELL, J.A., TURK, J.L. and BAKER, D., 1989, Regulation of lymphocyte proliferation in contact sensitivity: homeostatic mechanisms and a possible explanation of antigenic competition, *Immunology*, **66**, 577–82.

KINNAIRD, A., PETERS, S.W., FOSTER, J.R. and KIMBER, I., 1989, Dendritic cell accumulation in draining lymph nodes during the induction phase of contact allergy in mice, *International Archives of Allergy and Applied Immunology*, **89**, 202–10.

KLEIJMEER, M.J., OORSCHOT, V.M.J. and GEUZE, H.J., 1994, Human resident Langerhans cells display a lysosomal compartment enriched in MHC class II, *Journal of Investigative Dermatology*, **103**, 516–23.

KNIGHT, S.C., KREJCI, J., MALKOVSKY, M., COLIZZI, V., GAUTAM, A. and ASHERSON, G.L., 1985, The role of dendritic cells in the initiation of immune responses to contact sensitizers. I. In vivo exposure to antigen, *Cellular Immunology*, **94**, 427–34.

KOCH, F., HEUFLER, C., KAMPGEN, E., SCHNEEWEISS, D., BOCK, G. and SCHULER, G., 1990, Tumor necrosis factor alpha maintains the viability of murine epidermal Langerhans cells in culture but in contrast to granulocyte/macrophage colony-stimulating factor, does not induce their functional maturation, *Journal of Experimental Medicine*, **171**, 159–72.

KOHLER, J., MARTIN, S., PFLUGFELDER, U., RUH, H., VOLLMER, J. and WELTZIEN, H.U., 1995, Cross-reactive trinitrophenylated peptides as antigens for class II major histocompatibility complex-restricted T cells and inducers of contact sensitivity in mice. Limited T cell receptor repertoire, *European Journal of Immunology*, **25**, 92–101.

KONDO, S., MCKENZIE, R.C. and SAUDER, D.N., 1994, Interleukin-10 inhibits the elicitation phase of allergic contact hypersensitivity, *Journal of Investigative Dermatology*, **103**, 811–4.

KONING, F., STINGL, G., YOKOYAMA, W.M., YAMADA, H., MALOY, W.L., TSCHACHLER, E., SHEVACH, E.M. and COLIGAN, J.E., 1987, Identification of T3-associated gamma-delta T cell receptor on Thy-1[+] dendritic epidermal cell lines, *Science*, **236**, 834–7.

KRIPKE, M.L., MUNN, C.G., JEEVAN, A., TANG, J-M. and BUCANA, C., 1990, Evidence that cutaneous antigen-presenting cells migrate to regional lymph nodes during contact sensitization, *Journal of Immunology*, **145**, 2833–8.

LARSEN, C.P., RITCHIE, S.C., PEARSON, T.C., LINSLEY, P.S. and LOWRY, R.P., 1992, Functional expression of the costimulatory molecule, B7/BB1, on murine dendritic cell populations, *Journal of Experimental Medicine*, **176**, 1215–20.

LE GROS, G. and ERARD, F., 1994, Non-cytotoxic, IL-4, IL-5, IL-10 producing

CD8$^+$ T cells: their activation and effector functions, *Current Opinion in Immunology*, **6**, 453–7.

LENZ, A., HEINE, M., SCHULER, G. and ROMANI, N., 1993, Human and murine dermis contain dendritic cells. Isolation by means of a novel method and phenotypical and functional characterization, *Journal of Clinical Investigation*, **93**, 2587–96.

LI, L., ELLIOTT, J.F. and MOSMANN, T.R., 1994, IL-10 inhibits cytokine production, vascular leakage and swelling during T helper 1 cell-induced delayed-type hypersensitivity, *Journal of Immunology*, **153**, 3967–78.

LOVE-SCHIMENTI, C.D. and KRIPKE, M.L., 1994, Dendritic epidermal T cells inhibit T lymphocyte proliferation and may induce tolerance by cytotoxicity, *Journal of Immunology*, **153**, 3450–6.

MA, J., WANG, J-H., GUO, Y-J., SY, M-S. and BIGBY, M., 1994, In vivo treatment with anti-ICAM-1 and anti-LFA-1 antibodies inhibits contact sensitization-induced migration of epidermal Langerhans cells to regional lymph nodes, *Cellular Immunology*, **158**, 389–99.

MACATONIA, S.E., DOHERTY, T.M., KNIGHT, S.C. and O'GARRA, A., 1993, Differential effect of IL-10 on dendritic cell-induced T cell proliferation and IFN-γ production, *Journal of Immunology*, **150**, 3755–65.

MACATONIA, S.E., EDWARDS, A.J. and KNIGHT, S.C., 1986, Dendritic cells and the initiation of contact sensitivity to fluorescein isothiocyanate, *Immunology*, **59**, 509–14.

MACATONIA, S.E. and KNIGHT, S.C., 1989, Dendritic cells and T cells transfer sensitization for delayed-type hypersensitivity after skin painting with contact sensitizer, *Immunology*, **66**, 96–9.

MACATONIA, S.E., KNIGHT, S.C., EDWARDS, A.J., GRIFFITHS, S. and FRYER, P., 1987, Localization of antigen on lymph node dendritic cells after exposure to the contact sensitizer fluorescein isothiocyanate. Functional and morphological studies, *Journal of Experimental Medicine*, **166**, 1654–67.

MAGUIRE, H.C. Jr., 1995, Murine recombinant interleukin-12 increases the acquisition of allergic contact dermatitis in the mouse, *International Archives of Allergy and Immunology*, **106**, 166–8.

MANETTI, R., PARRONCHI, P., GIUDIZI, M.G., PICCINNI, M-P., MAGGI, G., TRINCHIERI, G. and ROMAGNANI, S., 1993, Natural killer cell stimulatory factor (interleukin 12 (IL-12)) induces T helper type 1 (Th1)-specific immune responses and inhibits the development of IL-4 producing Th cells, *Journal of Experimental Medicine*, **177**, 1199–204.

MARKEY, A.C., ALLEN, M.H., PITZALIS, C. and MACDONALD, D.M., 1990, T-cell inducer populations in cutaneous inflammation: a predominance of T-helper-inducer lymphocytes in the infiltrate of inflammatory dermatoses, *British Journal of Dermatology*, **122**, 325–32.

MATSUE, H., CRUZ, P.D. Jr., BERGSTRESSER, P.R. and TAKASHIMA, A., 1992, Langerhans cells are the major source of mRNA for IL-1β and MIP-1α among unstimulated mouse epidermal cells, *Journal of Investigative Dermatology*, **99**, 537–41.

MCKENZIE, R.C. and SAUDER, D.N., 1990, The role of keratinocyte cytokines in inflammation and immunity, *Journal of Investigative Dermatology*, **95**, 105S-107S.

MOSMANN, T.R., CHERWINSKI, H., BOND, M.W., GEIDLIN, M.A. and COF-

FMAN, R.L., 1986, Two types of murine helper T cell clone. 1. Definition according to lymphokine activities and secreted proteins, *Journal of Immunology*, **136**, 2348–57.

MOSMANN, T.R. and COFFMAN, R.L., 1989, Heterogeneity of cytokine secretion patterns and functions of T helper cells, *Advances in Immunology*, **46**, 111–47.

MOSMANN, T.R., SCHUMACHER, J.H., STREET, N.F., BUDD, R., O'GARRA, A., FONG, T.A.T., BOND, M.W., MOORE, K.W.M., SHER, A. and FIORENTINO, D.F., 1991, Diversity of cytokine synthesis and function of mouse CD4$^+$ T cells, *Immunological Reviews*, **123**, 209–29.

NESTLE, F.O., ZHENG, X-G., THOMPSON, C.B., TURKA, L.A. and NICKOLOFF, B.J., 1993, Characterization of dermal dendritic cells obtained from normal human skin reveals phenotypic and functionally distinct subsets, *Journal of Immunology*, **151**, 6535–45.

OHMEN, J.D., HANIFIN, J.M., NICKOLOFF, B.J., REA, T.H., WYZYKOWSKI, R., KIM, J., JULLIEN, D., MCHUGH, T., NASSIF, A.S., CHAN, S.C. and MODLIN, R.L., 1995, Overexpression of IL-10 in atopic dermatitis. Contrasting cytokine patterns with delayed-type hypersensitivity reactions, *Journal of Immunology*, **154**, 1956–63.

PEGUET-NAVARRO, J., MOULON, C., CAUX, C., DALBIEZ-GAUTHIER, C., BANCHEREAU, J. and SCHMITT, D., 1994, Interleukin-10 inhibits the primary allogeneic T cell response to human epidermal Langerhans cells, *European Journal of Immunology*, **24**, 884–91.

PICKER, L.J., KISHIMOTO, T.K., SMITH, C.W., WARNOCK, R.A. and BUTCHER, E.C., 1991, ELAM-1 is an adhesion molecule for skin-homing T cells, *Nature*, **349**, 796–9.

PICKER, L.J., MICHIE, S.A., ROTT, L.S. and BUTCHER, E.C., 1990, A unique phenotype of skin-associated lymphocytes in humans, *American Journal of Pathology*, **136**, 1053–68.

PICKER, L.J., TREER, J.R., FERGUSON-DARNELL, B., COLLINS, P.A., BERGSTRESSER, P.R. and TERSTAPPEN, L.W.M.M., 1993, Control of lymphocyte recirculation in man. II. Differential regulation of cutaneous lymphocyte-associated antigen, a tissue-selective homing receptor for skin-homing T cells, *Journal of Immunology*, **150**, 1122–36.

PICUT, C.A., LEE, C.S., DOUGHERTY, E.P., ANDERSON, K.L. and LEWIS, R.M., 1988, Immunostimulatory capabilities of highly enriched Langerhans cells in vitro, *Journal of Investigative Dermatology*, **90**, 201–6.

RAZI-WOLF, Z., FALO, L.D. Jr. and REISER, H., 1994, Expression and function of the costimulatory molecule B7 on murine Langerhans cells: evidence for an alternative CTLA-4 ligand, *European Journal of Immunology*, **24**, 805–11.

REIS E SOUSA, C., STAHL, P.D. and AUSTYN, J.M., 1993, Phagocytosis of antigens by Langerhans cells in vitro, *Journal of Experimental Medicine*, **178**, 509–19.

ROBINSON, D., HAMID, Q., BENTLEY, A., YING, S., KAY, A.B. and DURHAM, S.R., 1993, Activation of CD4$^+$ T cells, increased T$_{H2}$-type cytokine mRNA expression and eosinophil recruitment in bronchoalveolar lavage after allergen inhalation challenge in patients with atopic asthma, *Journal of Allergy and Clinical Immunology*, **92**, 313–24.

ROBINSON, D.S., HAMID, Q., YING, S., TSICHPOULOS, A., BARKANS, J., BENTLEY, A.M., CORRIGAN, C., DURHAM, S.R. and KAY, A.B., 1992,

Predominant T_{H2}-like bronchoalveolar T-lymphocyte population in atopic asthma, *The New England Journal of Medicine*, **326**, 298–304.

ROBINSON, M.K, 1989, Optimization of an in vitro lymphocyte blastogenesis assay for predictive assessment of immunologic responsiveness to contact sensitizers, *Journal of Investigative Dermatology*, **92**, 860–7.

ROMAGNANI, S., 1991, Human T_{H1} and T_{H2} subsets: doubt no more, *Immunology Today*, **12**, 256–7.

ROMAGNANI, S., 1992, Induction of T_{H1} and T_{H2} responses : a key role for the 'natural' immune response?, *Immunology Today*, **13**, 379–81.

ROMAGNANI, S., DEL PRETE, B., MAGGI, E., PARRONCHI, P., DE CARLI, M., MACCHIA, D., MANETTI, R., SAMPOGNARO, S., PICCINNI, M-P., GIUDIZI, M.G., BIAGIOTTI, R. and ALMERIGOGNA, F., 1992, Human T_{H1} and T_{H2} subsets, *International Archives of Allergy and Immunology*, **99**, 242–5.

SAITO, S., DORF, M.E., WATANABE, N. and TADAKUMA, T., 1994, Preferential induction of IL-4 is determined by the type and duration of antigenic stimulation, *Cellular Immunology*, **153**, 1–8.

SALERNO, A., DIELI, F., SIRECI, G., BELLAVIA, A. and ASHERSON, G.L., 1995, Interleukin-4 is a critical cytokine in contact sensitivity, *Immunology*, **84**, 404–9.

SANTAMARIA BABI, L.F., MOSER, R., PEREZ SOLER, M.F., PICKER, L.J., BLASER, K. and HAUSER, C., 1995, Migration of skin-homing T cells across cytokine-activated human endothelial cell layers involves interaction of the cutaneous lymphocyte-associated antigen (CLA), the very late antigen-4 (VLA-4) and the lymphocyte function-associated antigen-1 (LFA-1), *Journal of Immunology*, **154**, 1543–50.

SCHMITT, E., HOEHN, P., HUELS, C., GOEDERT, S., PALM, N., RUDE, E. and GERMANN, T., 1994, T helper type 1 development of naive CD4[+] T cells requires the coordinate action of interleukin-12 and interferon-γ and is inhibited by transforming growth factor-β, *European Journal of Immunology*, **24**, 793–8.

SCHREIBER, S., KILGUS, O., PAYER, E., KUTIL, R., ELBE, A., MUELLER, C. and STINGL, G., 1992, Cytokine pattern of Langerhans cells isolated from murine epidermal cell cultures, *Journal of Immunology*, **149**, 3525–34.

SCHULER and STEINMAN, R.M., 1985, Murine epidermal Langerhans cells mature into potent immunostimulatory dendritic cells in vitro, *Journal of Experimental Medicine*, **161**, 526–46.

SHELLEY, W.B. and JUHLIN, L., 1976, Langerhans cells form a reticuloepithelial trap for external contact allergens, *Nature*, **261**, 46–7.

SILBER, A., NEWMAN, W., SASSEVILLE, V.G., PAULEY, D., BEALL, D., WALSH, D.G. and RINGLER, D.J., 1994, Recruitment of lymphocytes during cutaneous delayed hypersensitivity in non-human primates is dependent on E-selectin and vascular cell adhesion molecule 1, *Journal of Clinical Investigation*, **93**, 1554–63.

SILVENNOINEN-KASSINEN, S., IKAHEIMO, I., KARVONEN, J., KAUPPINEN, M. and KALLIOINEN, M., 1992, Mononuclear cell subsets in the nickel allergic reaction in vitro and in vivo, *Journal of Allergy and Applied Immunology*, **89**, 794–800.

SINIGAGLIA, F., 1994, The molecular basis of metal recognition by T cells, *Journal of Investigative Dermatology*, **102**, 398–401.

STREILEIN, J.W. and GRAMMER, S.F., 1989, In vitro evidence that Langerhans cells can adopt two functionally distinct forms capable of antigen presentation to T lymphocytes, *Journal of Immunology*, **143**, 3925–33.

STREILEIN, J.W., GRAMMER, S.F., YOSHIKAWA, T., DEMIDEM, A. and VERMEER, M., 1990, Functional dichotomy between Langerhans cells that present antigen to naive and memory/effector T lymphocytes, *Immunological Reviews*, **117**, 159–83.

SULLIVAN, S., BERGSTRESSER, P.R., TIGELAAR, R.E. and STREILEIN, J.W., 1986, Induction and regulation of contact hypersensitivity by resident bone marrow-derived dendritic epidermal cells. Langerhans cells and Thy-1$^+$ epidermal cells, *Journal of Immunology*, **137**, 2460–7.

SWAIN, S.L., BRADLEY, L.M., CROFT, M., TONKONOGY, S., ATKINS, G., WEINBERG, A.D., DUNCAN, D.D., HEDRICK, S.M., DUTTEN, R.W. and HUSTON, G., 1991, Helper T-cell subsets: phenotype, function and the role of lymphokines in regulating their development, *Immunological Reviews*, **123**, 115–44.

TANG, A., AMAGAI, M., GRANGER, L.G., STANLEY, J.R. and UDEY, M.C., 1993, Adhesion of epidermal Langerhans cells to keratinocytes mediated by E-cadherin, *Nature*, **361**, 82–5.

TREDE, N.S., GEHA, R.S. and CHATILA, T., 1991, Transcriptional activation of IL-1β and tumor necrosis factor-α genes by MHC class II ligands, *Journal of Immunology*, **146**, 2310–5.

TRINCHIERI, G., 1994, Interleukin-12 and its role in the generation of Th-1 cells, *Immunology Today*, **14**, 335–7.

TSCHACHLER, E., SCHULER, G., HUTTERER, J., LEIBL, H., WOLFF, K. and STINGL, G., 1983, Expression of Thy-1 antigen by murine epidermal dendritic cells, *Journal of Investigative Dermatology*, **81**, 282–5.

TSE, Y. and COOPER, K.D., 1990, Cutaneous dermal Ia$^+$ cells are capable of initiating delayed-type hypersensitivity responses, *Journal of Investigative Dermatology*, **94**, 267–72.

VAN DER HEIJDEN, F.L., WIERENGA, E.A., BOS, J.D. and KAPSENBERG, M.L., 1991, High frequency of IL-4-producing CD4$^+$ allergen-specific T lymphocytes in atopic dermatitis lesional skin, *Journal of Investigative Dermatology*, **97**, 389–94.

WEAVER, C.T., HAWRYLOWICZ, C.M. and UNANUE, E.R., 1988, T helper cell subsets require the expression of distinct costimulatory signals by antigen-presenting cells, *Proceedings of the National Academy of Sciences, USA*, **85**, 8181–5.

WELSH, E.A. and KRIPKE, M.L., 1990, Murine Thy-1$^+$ dendritic epidermal cells induce immunologic tolerance in vivo, *Journal of Immunology*, **144**, 883–91.

WHITE, S.I., FRIEDMANN, P.S., MOSS, C. and SIMPSON, J.M., 1986, The effect of altering area of application and dose per unit area on sensitization by DNCB, *British Journal of Dermatology*, **115**, 663–8.

WINZEN, R., WALLACH, D., KEMPER, O., RESCH, K. and HOLTMANN, H., 1993, Selective up-regulation of the 75-kDa tumor necrosis factor (TNF) receptor and its mRNA by TNF and IL-1, *Journal of Immunology*, **150**, 4346–53.

WITMER-PACK, M.D., OLIVIER, W., VALINSKY, J., SCHULER, G. and STEINMAN, R.M., 1987, Granulocyte/macrophage colony-stimulating factor is essential for the viability and function of cultured murine epidermal Langerhans cells, *Journal of Experimental Medicine*, **166**, 1484–98.

3

Clinical Aspects of Allergic Contact Dermatitis

P.S. FRIEDMANN

Royal Liverpool University Hospital

Introduction

One of the major functions of skin is the provision of a protective barrier defending the body against noxious agents in the environment. The barrier has to be maintained by continued self renewal and repair of breaches caused by injury. The physical properties of stratum corneum limit the passage of water, electrolytes and many chemical substances. The epidermis functions as a physical barrier against invasion by microbes. However, the skin is more than a passive barricade – it has to play an active role, responding to perturbations, whether physical or chemical, by actively recruiting inflammatory mechanisms which can include specific components of the immune system. The involvement of the skin in immune defence is particularly important in relation to microbes that penetrate into the epidermis, such as viruses, fungi and parasites, including the scabies mite. In responding to chemical perturbations the skin cannot distinguish between microbial products and other environmentally derived substances. If the substance is immunogenic the immune system is activated and the response evoked by chemicals/antigens from microbes may be indistinguishable from that induced by non-microbial haptens – so-called contact sensitizers. The result is a delayed-type hypersensitivity characterized by the infiltration of CD4$^+$ T lymphocytes into both dermis and epidermis. Experimental contact hypersensitivity has been used to elucidate mechanisms involved in the immune response both regarding the induction of sensitization, the afferent limb, and also the expression of the immune response in the efferent limb.

26

The Clinical Problem of Contact Hypersensitivity

Immune responses to microbes that penetrate into the viable layers of epidermis are recognized clinically as "eczema". Thus, fungal infection of the feet may result in a vesicular foot eczema, whilst infestation with scabies mites induces a diffuse eczematous reaction with local concentrations in the finger webs. The immune/allergic response to environmental sensitizers results in the inflammatory reaction of allergic contact eczema or dermatitis. This often happens as an unwanted consequence of exposure to substances in the domestic or work environments. Contact with the provoking agent results in a characteristic distribution of the inflammation (Figure 3.1). Underlying the inflammation is vasodilatation resulting in redness (erythema) and increased vascular permeability with formation of oedema causing swelling and induration. In addition, oedema forms within the epidermis, separating epidermal cells – called spongiosis – and forming vesicles which, when large, can be seen to be multilocular because of the fusion of small vesicles. There is perivascular inflammatory infiltration of lymphomononuclear cells in the dermis. The most important component is probably CD4$^+$ T cells which are also found in the epidermis (for more details see below). Allergic contact dermatitis is recognized clinically from the anatomical distribution of lesions in areas matching physical contact with likely provoking agents in the environment. The picture can become confused because many chemical substances can act as irritants, provoking inflammatory reactions which are not mediated by specific immune mechanisms. Reactions to irritants are classified as acute when they follow a single exposure to the substance or chronic when they result from repeated or cumulative exposure to the provoking compounds. Responses to irritants must be mentioned here because, as will be seen later, certain mechanisms are common to both the non-immune and immune mediated processes. The presence of specific lymphocyte mediated immune reactivity is demonstrated by epicutaneous patch test challenge with the relevant substance. The inflammatory response develops over 24–48 hours and may last up to a week. The crucial aspect of the patch test technique is the concentration of antigen which must be below the level that causes irritancy. This is essential to avoid elicitation of non-specific inflammatory responses.

Incidence and Prevalence of Allergic Contact Dermatitis

Estimation of incidence and prevalence of contact dermatitis in a whole population is very difficult. A number of surveys have been performed and most have been cross-sectional, that is they have looked at a population sample that is presumed to represent the general population with no selection in relation to exposure or disease status. Most studies have used questionnaires, asking for the presence of skin troubles on the hands, and most

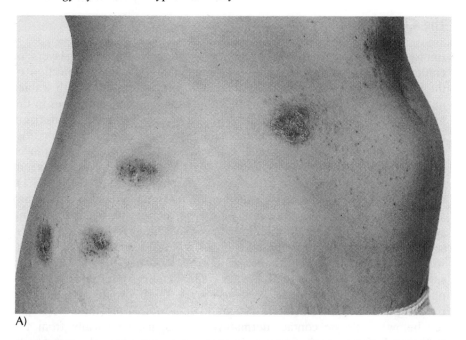

A)

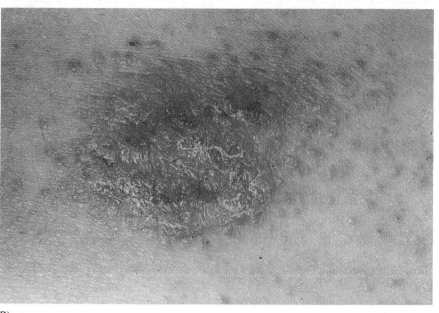

B)

Figure 3.1 A) Clinical appearance of allergic contact dermatitis. The lesions correspond to sites of contact with the nickel in jean's studs. B) Close up of one patch to show the classical appearance of eczema. The lesion has edges that break up into small papules – the minimal lesion of eczema

followed up with a clinical examination to confirm responses to the questionnaires. These have mainly given estimates for the occurrence of eczema without distinction between irritant or allergic contact dermatitis. Figures for the prevalence of hand dermatitis include:

1.7% in Sweden (Agrup, 1969)
6.3% in Sweden (Meding and Swanbeck, 1987)
8.9% in Norway (Kavli and Forde, 1984)
2% in the USA (Johnson and Roberts, 1978)
6.1% in London (Rea *et al.*, 1976).

For the detailed summary of these surveys see Mathias (1985).

In the working population of the western world, occupational skin disease accounts for about one-third of all chronic occupational diseases. Eczema and contact dermatitis are responsible for 85–95 per cent of all causes of occupational skin diseases (Emmet, 1984; Mathias, 1985).

Exposure to sensitizing substances is obviously a prerequisite for the formation of allergic contact sensitivity, but, given comparable exposure, there are a number of factors that contribute to whether and how sensitivity is manifest.

Studies of Susceptibility to Contact Sensitization

The generation of an immune response involves two distinct components – the initiation of sensitization, the afferent limb, and the expression of the sensitivity once it is established, the efferent limb. Both these components of the response are influenced by systemic factors including genetic constitution, age and sex as well as local factors including regional differences in skin thickness, barrier function, vasculature and perhaps many others. Many attempts have been made to examine the importance of these in determining immune responsiveness.

What determines whether an individual will develop an immune/ hypersensitivity response to a substance? Antigenic strength or potency is still not well understood, but some substances such as dinitrochlorobenzene (DNCB), diphenylcyclopropenone (DPCP), oxazolone and urushiol (poison ivy) are highly potent and appear able to induce sensitization in all normal people. Substances such as metallic salts of nickel, cobalt and chromium, or a huge range of organic compounds, are weak antigens and appear only to sensitize some subjects. It is not known whether every individual has the capacity to respond to weak sensitizers. The concentration of antigen is critical and local factors that potentiate percutaneous absorption, such as occlusion or coincident inflammation, may augment the sensitizing potency of a substance. An additional factor that is not yet widely recognized is the capacity to metabolize xenobiotics in ways that may generate reactive or antigenic intermediates. Indirect evidence suggests that phenotype for glutathione S-transferase, which metabolizes DNCB, could be one such determinant of sensitivity (de Berker *et al.*, 1995).

Once a substance penetrates the outer barrier of the stratum corneum, the induction of sensitization is mediated by specialized antigen-presenting cells – Langerhans cells (LC). In summary, upon contact with a chemical, LC in the epidermis descend into the dermis and migrate via the afferent lymphatics to the regional lymph node. Here, they enter the paracortical areas, the home of T lymphocytes (Macatonia *et al.*, 1986; Okamoto and Kripe, 1987; Kinnaird *et al.*, 1989). If the substance is an antigen it appears to provoke this migration. Also, the LC expresses the substance on its surface in combination with the class II molecules of the major histocompatibility complex (MHC), HLA-DR in humans. This complex of HLA-DR associated with antigen is recognized by a T lymphocyte expressing the appropriate specific T cell receptor. The specific receptor-mediated binding with the antigen-bearing Langerhans cell causes activation of the T cell resulting in proliferation and expansion of the clone to establish a population of CD4$^+$ effector T cells. These processes are considered in detail in Chapter 2.

Once some degree of clonal expansion has occurred, immunological "memory" is established and, upon re-encounter with the antigen, a quicker response is mobilized. If the clonal expansion continues, at some point some of the daughter cells will leave the node to enter the circulation. Once in the circulation they are available to participate in immune surveillance and to traffic through the tissues. Their presence is manifested by the inflammatory response of allergic contact eczema which develops at sites of encounter with their specific antigen. The regulation of many steps in these events are not yet understood. For instance, what determines how many initial T cells are encountered by the antigen-bearing Langerhans cells, or how many divisions the expanding T cell clone undergoes? What signals some T cells to leave the node? What contributes to the generation of the inflammatory response in the efferent stage? It is variability in these steps that probably accounts for the heterogeneity of immune responsiveness seen in human beings. However, despite the many steps that are involved in the generation of an immune response, the human immune system, like other physiological systems, exhibits tidy and generally predictable dose-response relationships. Using experimental sensitization with DNCB, analysis of these dose-response relationships has given a physiological perspective to many of the static and qualitative phenomena observed experimentally.

Experimental Sensitization with DNCB

DNCB is a highly potent contact sensitizer and has been used for many studies of human immune responses (Rostenberg and Kanof, 1941; Epstein and Maibach, 1965; Eilber and Morton, 1970; Catalona *et al.*, 1972; Bleumink *et al.*, 1974; Friedmann *et al.*, 1983; de Berker *et al.*, 1995). The author and colleagues examined the effects of varying the sensitizing dose of DNCB on contact sensitization, and also the dose-response relationships of the elicitation reaction (Friedmann *et al.*, 1983; Friedmann and Moss, 1985; Friedmann, 1986). Five groups of normal subjects, with no history of contact sensitivity or inflammatory skin disease, received sensitizing doses of 62.5, 125, 250, 500 or 1000 μg of DNCB in acetone. The sensitizing dose was applied to the flexor aspect of the forearm on a standard, 3 cm diameter area, followed by occlusion for 48 hours. Some DNCB remains bound in the skin for several weeks and hence is available to act as a continuous challenge. As soon as the DNCB-specific T cells enter the circulation they can respond to this challenge generating inflammation at the site – a reaction which has been called the "delayed flare" by earlier workers. It was observed that the time of onset of this reaction was inversely related to sensitizing dose (Figure 3.2). This implied that the clonal expansion had been quicker which suggests that a greater number of cells had been activated at the outset.

Four weeks after induction of sensitization a graded series of challenges – 3.125, 6.25, 12.5 and 25 μg – were applied to the other forearm on standard 1 cm patch test felts (A1-test) for 24 hours. Forty-eight hours after application the responses were measured with Harpenden calipers as increase in skin fold thickness (Friedmann *et al.*, 1983).

DNCB is an irritant, so in order to interpret challenge responses the irritant effect was first examined in unsensitized normal subjects. The irritant reaction was mainly one of erythema and not oedema (Figure 3.3). Within the range of challenge doses studied the threshold for irritancy was 25 μg and there was little further increase in thickness at higher challenge doses. Hence, the small degree of thickness change due to irritancy was assumed to be constant and not to contribute significantly to the specific immune reaction. Because of the problem of detecting a degree of reactivity so low it could only be elicited by challenge doses above the threshold for irritancy, subjects with no response below this 25 μg dose were regarded, arbitrarily, as unsensitized. Using the clinical assessment of an indurated (oedematous) response to challenge with 12.5 μg to indicate that sensitivity was detectable, it was found that the proportions of subjects sensitized showed a sigmoid relationship with the log of sensitizing dose (Figure 3.4). Thus, 100 per cent of people were sensitized by an initial application of 500 μg of DNCB. When the sigmoid log dose-response curve was linearized by logit transformation, the dose required to sensitize 50 per cent of subjects (ED_{50}) was estimated as 116 μg. This was subsequently tested, and indeed 13 of 26 subjects were sensitized (Friedmann *et al.*, 1990).

The data obtained from these five groups raised the question of how strength of sensitizing stimulus affected degree of reactivity. It was observed that as sensitizing dose increased, not only were more people made clinically sensitive, they were sensitized to a greater degree. Challenge of these five groups produced a family of dose-response curves that appear to be the lower portions of sigmoid curves (Figure 3.3). The tops of the curves were not

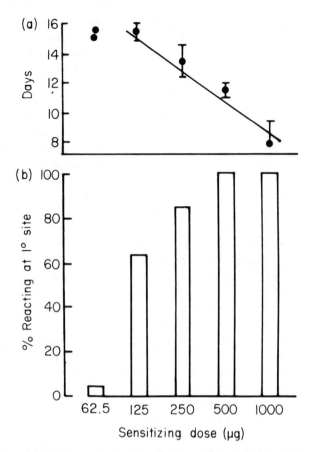

Figure 3.2 "Late" flare reaction at site of primary sensitization with DNCB.
a) Time of appearance of reaction. b) Proportion of subjects developing such
reactions with different sensitizing doses. (Reproduced with permission from
Friedmann, *Clinical & Experimental Dermatology*, 1991)

reached within the range of doses used. Analysis of the linear portions
confirmed they were parallel and the calculated slopes are shown in Figure
3.5. It can be seen that as sensitizing dose increases so the challenge dose-
response curve is shifted progressively to the left indicating greater reactivity.

The fact that changing the strength of the sensitizing stimulus altered the
position of the dose-response curve, but not its slope, is informative. The
slope of the curve seems likely to be determined by the local inflammatory
response, the increments of change being proportional to the log of the
eliciting stimulus. The position of the challenge dose-response curve reflects
the "degree of sensitivity" of an individual or group of subjects. Since the
curves are parallel, they can be represented by the responses at any challenge

RESPONSE TO CHALLENGE WITH DNCB

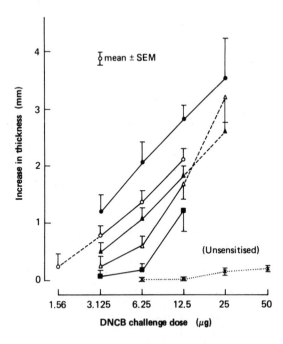

Figure 3.3 Response to challenge with DNCB in subjects challenged with different doses of DNCB. ● = Sensitizing dose (SD) 1000 μg, ○ = SD 500 μg, ▲ = SD 250 μg, △ = SD 125 μg, ■ = 62.5 μg, X = unsensitized controls to show irritant effect. Responses measured with calipers as skin fold thickness. Dashed lines are data from few subjects. (Reproduced with permission from Friedmann *et al.*, 1983)

dose. Thus, when the response at the 12.5 μg challenge dose for each group of subjects is plotted against the sensitizing dose, a curve is obtained which shows that as sensitizing stimulus increases so there is a uniform, linear augmentation of degree of sensitivity (Figure 3.6). This probably reflects the proliferative expansion of a clone or clones of antigen-specific effector T cells, or conceivably of both T effector and T suppressor cells. However, in the latter case their net contribution would have to increase uniformly. The slope of the curve in Figure 3.6 which reflects increase in sensitivity with increasing sensitizing dose, reflects the contribution of regulatory factors, augmenting or "helper" factors being likely to increase the slope, while inhibitory or "suppressor" factors being likely to depress it. The slope of this curve, therefore, represents the "susceptibility" to contact sensitization by DNCB in normal subjects. The slope of the curve would be expected to alter with disease or treatment that modifies susceptibility.

33

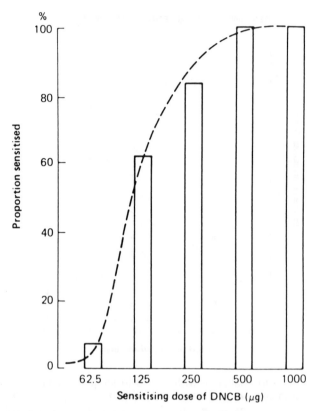

Figure 3.4 Proportion of normal subjects sensitized by different doses of DNCB. (Reproduced with permission from Friedmann and Moss, 1985)

Variation in Susceptibility to Contact Sensitization

There is considerable variation in susceptibility to contact sensitization even among people who appear "normal" in every sense. Thus, at any sensitizing dose below the 100 per cent effective dose – for example 250 μg – of those who gave clinically "positive" reactions to the challenges there was a very wide range of responses which appeared normally distributed. However, a proportion of people appeared not to be sensitized at all. The question that arises from this is what has happened immunologically in these unresponsive subjects? Was it a complete failure of response or has their immune system responded to the stimulus at a sub-clinical level? If this were the case it would be expected that the initial sensitizing dose has in fact primed the system, initiating expansion of the specifically committed clone(s) to establish some degree of immunological memory. From this it might be predicted that a second sensitizing stimulus would induce an augmented or boosted response.

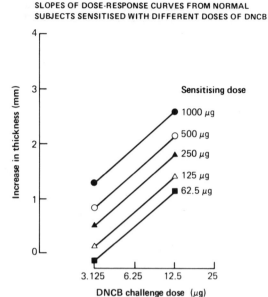

SLOPES OF DOSE-RESPONSE CURVES FROM NORMAL
SUBJECTS SENSITISED WITH DIFFERENT DOSES OF DNCB

Figure 3.5 Responses to challenge with DNCB in normal subjects sensitized 4 weeks previously. The calculated slopes of the linear portions of dose response curves are shown. (Reproduced with permission from Friedmann and Moss, 1985)

This is in fact the case as shown by the following observations. The approach employed to test the possibility made use of the fact that the challenge regimen of 4 DNCB doses (3.125, 6.25, 12.5 and 25 μg; total 46.9 μg) is itself a moderately potent sensitizing stimulus. Thus, the degree of reactivity of control subjects sensitized by application of the challenge regimen alone could be determined with a second, elicitation challenge, 4 weeks after the first sensitizing exposure (Figure 3.7). Responses could be compared with those from subjects given the same regimen but who had first received a low potency sensitizing stimulus. Therefore, a group of normal people received 116 μg DNCB on a 3 cm circle of forearm skin as initial sensitizing stimulus. This had previously been shown to be the 50 per cent effective sensitizing dose (Friedmann *et al.*, 1990). When challenged 4 weeks later, half the subjects showed no clinically detectable response. These unresponsive subjects were challenged a second time after 4 more weeks (Figure 3.7). They gave greatly augmented responses compared with the control subjects who 4 weeks previously had received the challenge regimen alone as a sensitizing stimulus (Figure 3.8). This showed clearly that the two sensitizing stimuli had interacted positively, the first sub-clinical stimulus having established immunological memory which greatly augmented the response to the second sensitizing stimulus. This experiment was repeated using the 25 per cent

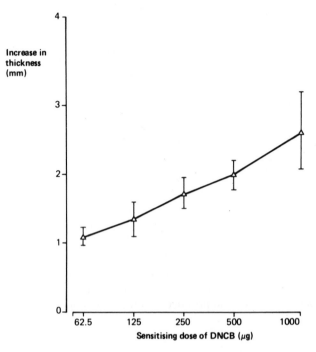

**NORMAL AUGMENTATION OF RESPONSIVENESS
WITH INCREASING SENSITISING DOSE OF DNCB**

Figure 3.6 Relationship between "degree of sensitization" and sensitizing dose. The skin fold thickness responses to challenge with 12.5 μg of DNCB from each group of subjects is plotted against sensitizing dose. Data from 5 groups of healthy subjects shown in Figure 3.5. (Bars are SEM) (Reproduced with permission from Friedmann and Moss, 1985)

effective sensitizing dose (75 μg DNCB) as the sub-clinical priming dose (Friedmann *et al.*, 1990). Again, the subjects who were unresponsive to the first elicitation challenge were given a second challenge after a further 4 weeks. These people were significantly more responsive than the controls and hence had clearly been sensitized at a sub-clinical level by the primary sensitizing dose (Friedmann *et al.*, 1990).

Thus, it is clear that a state of sub-clinical sensitization can be established by exposure to low dose of antigen. This indicates therefore that the quantitative dose relationship of contact sensitization by DNCB extends down into the sub-clinical range. This fits with the clonal expansion of antigen-specific T lymphocytes but supports the idea that below certain levels of proliferation, these cells remain within the lymph nodes and cannot participate in cutaneous challenge responses.

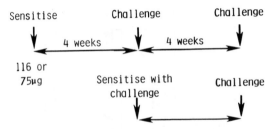

Figure 3.7 Protocol for sensitization and challenge to assess sub-clinical sensitization. Experimental subjects received an initial dose of 116 or 75 μg of DNCB. Four weeks later they were challenged and subjects who were unresponsive received a further challenge after 4 more weeks. Control subjects received the challenge regimen to induce sensitization and their degree of reactivity was determined 4 weeks later with an eliciting challenge. (Reproduced from Friedmann *et al.*, 1990, with permission)

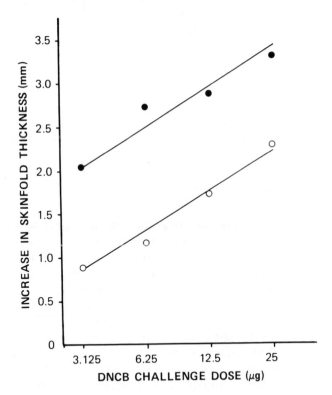

Figure 3.8 Augmentation of responsiveness by "sub-clinical" sensitization. After an initial dose of 116 μg of DNCB subjects were challenged 4 weeks later. Unresponsive subjects received a second challenge to determine their degree of reactivity (●). Control subjects were sensitized by application of the challenge regimen. (○). (Reproduced from Friedmann *et al.*, 1990, with permission)

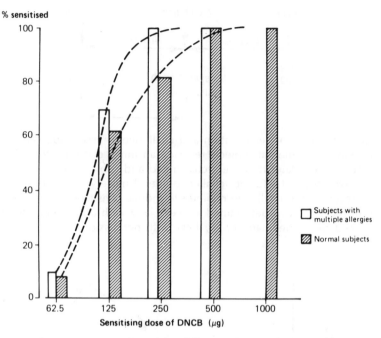

Figure 3.9 Proportions sensitized by different doses of DNCB. Comparison of normal subjects, as in Figure 3.4, with four groups of individuals with multiple contact allergies to environmental sensitizers. (Reproduced from Friedmann and Thody, 1986, with permission)

High Responders

It is a clinical observation that some individuals appear to form contact sensitivities readily to a wide range of environmental substances. This group was studied to see whether they were different in their capacity to respond to DNCB. Subjects with sensitivity to three or more antigens in the European standard patch test battery were identified from the diagnostic patch test clinic; patients with active eczema were excluded. The protocol for sensitization with DNCB was as described except that 1000 μg was not used. It was found that at each sensitizing dose proportionally more subjects could be sensitized (Figure 3.9) and the 100 per cent sensitizing dose was 250 μg. The sensitized subjects were more responsive than "normal" subjects (Figure 3.10), the challenge dose-response curves being displaced upwards compared with those of the normal subjects (Friedmann *et al.*, 1983; Friedmann *et al.*, 1990). Very interestingly, the slopes of the curves were parallel, indicating the increased contact sensitivity was not simply due to an increased capacity to generate inflammatory reactions in skin.

When the curve is plotted showing the relationship between degree of sensitization and sensitizing dose for this group of people with multiple

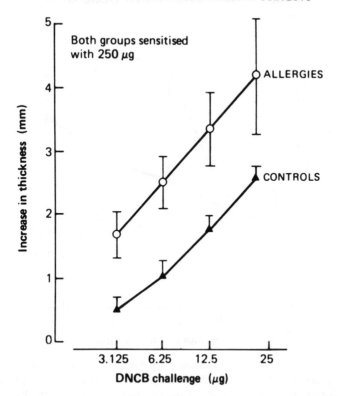

REACTIVITY TO DNCB OF SUBJECTS WITH MULTIPLE
ALLERGIES COMPARED WITH HEALTHY SUBJECTS

Figure 3.10 Responses to challenge with DNCB in subjects with multiple contact sensitivities (○) compared with those from normal subjects (▲). Data from subjects sensitized with 250 μg DNCB. (Reproduced from Friedmann and Thody, 1986, with permission)

contact sensitivities, it has a much greater slope than that for people without such allergies (Figure 3.11) (Friedmann, 1986). In other words, there is a greater augmentation of sensitivity produced by any increase in sensitizing dose.

One question that arises is whether the acquisition of one contact sensitivity increases susceptibility to further sensitization by other antigens. However, the studies by Moss *et al.* (1985) included some subjects with multiple contact sensitivities following occupational exposure. These subjects did not differ in their reactivity to DNCB suggesting that previous contact sensitivity *per se* does not enhance subsequent susceptibility to sensitization.

The subjects with multiple contact sensitivities might be a qualitatively different sub-group or they might be at one tail of the normal distribution. When people who had only a single contact sensitivity to nickel were tested with the same protocol, the slope of the curve for increasing sensitization

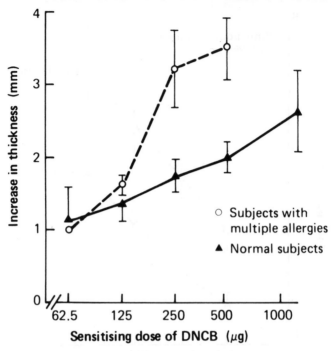

AUGMENTATION OF RESPONSIVENESS WITH INCREASING SENSITISING DOSE OF DNCB

Figure 3.11 Augmentation of sensitivity with increased sensitizing dose of DNCB. Degree of sensitization, obtained from response at 12.5 μg challenge dose, is plotted against sensitizing dose for normal subjects and those with multiple allergies. (Reproduced from Friedmann and Thody, 1986, with permission)

with sensitizing dose was intermediate (Moss *et al.*, 1985). There is evidence to support the idea that there is a normal distribution of susceptibility to contact sensitivities, "high responders" lying at one tail of the normal distribution, the other tail presumably being the "low responders".

Factors Influencing Susceptibility to Contact Sensitization

A number of studies have been performed to examine the basis of susceptibility to contact sensitivity.

Genetic Factors

Work in experimental animals provides many examples showing that genetic factors can be of major importance. Thus, inbred guinea pigs of strain II can be sensitized with chromate and beryllium but not mercury, whereas animals of strain XIII can be sensitized with mercury but not with chromate or beryllium (Polak *et al.*, 1968). In humans, naturally occurring sensitivity such as that to nickel and also deliberate experimental sensitization with chemicals has been observed. Walker *et al.* (1967) used two experimental sensitizers, DNCB and *p*-nitrosodimethylaniline (NDMA), to investigate responsiveness in families. It was found that if both parents could be sensitized by both agents then their children were more likely to be sensitized than were children whose parents failed to sensitize. However, it was not established whether this was simply quantitative in that they were less responsive but could have been sensitized by a bigger dose of antigen, or whether it was qualitative, that non-responders could not be sensitized at all. Work by the present author and colleagues suggests these would only be quantitative differences – that some humans are more susceptible to forming contact allergies (Friedmann,1989a; Friedmann *et al.*, 1990) (see above). In studies of female twins Menné and Holm (1983, 1986) found that among 30 pairs of monozygotic and 41 pairs of dizygotic twins with proven nickel allergy in one member of the pair, the frequency of hand eczema was 41 per cent in both groups. In monozygotic twins with one of the pair having nickel sensitivity, the chance of the other developing nickel sensitivity was comparable to the background population level – rather strong evidence against genetic control of susceptibility.

Several studies have examined whether susceptibility to contact sensitivity is linked to an HLA phenotype. In people with nickel sensitivity HLA DRw6 was found to be increased up to two-fold (37.7 per cent compared with 15.6 per cent in control subjects) (Menne and Holm, 1983). White *et al.* (1986b) examined 67 patients with multiple (three or more) independent contact allergies and found no overall HLA association with high susceptibility status. There was a small but non-significant increase in frequency of HLA-DR4 in subjects whose allergies included nickel, and of DR6 in those sensitized to rubber accelerators. Overall, apart from the report by Walker *et al.* (1967), there is very little to suggest that human susceptibility to contact hypersensitivity is under genetic control. One caveat, however, is that in all studies of HLA sensitization reviewed by the author, control populations were not screened to exclude the presence of contact sensitivity. Therefore, small differences may in fact be larger. Also, if human susceptibility to contact sensitivity is distributed normally, as indicated by the experimental studies with DNCB, then it is not surprising that there is no obvious link with HLA or other genetic factors.

Age

The ability to become sensitized to contact antigens such as DNCB changes very little with age (Schwartz, 1953; Friedmann *et al.*, 1983). The relationship between sensitizability and age showed no simple relationship although there

41

is a complex interaction between age and sex (Friedmann *et al.*, 1983). Thus, greatest responses were seen in young females, while lowest responses were obtained from old males (Friedmann *et al.*, 1983). Also, sensitizability is found to decline slightly after the age of 70.

A more important factor in relation to clinical problems from contact hypersensitivity is that with increasing age there is a greater chance of exposure to environmental allergens. Thus, the frequency of clinical problem of contact sensitization and positive patch tests increases with age at least up to the sixth decade.

Sex

Susceptibility to contact hypersensitivity is significantly greater in females. This is reflected by the fact that more females than males present with problems relating to contact hypersensitivity. In Newcastle upon Tyne (UK) analysis of results of patch tests with the European Standard Battery of antigens, performed over 5 years in nearly 2200 consecutive patients with eczema, showed the ratio of females to males with at least one positive patch test was > 3:1 (Moss, 1983). However, this might reflect either a fundamental sex difference or differences in environmental exposure to antigens.

A number of studies have examined susceptibility to contact hypersensitivity formally. Most have used experimental sensitization in different ways and have used response to challenge to make the qualitative decision as to whether an individual is sensitized or not. Walker *et al.* (1967) used DNCB, Leyden and Kligman (1977) and Jordan and King (1977) used repetitive exposure to panels of several antigens; all found small increases in the proportion of females becoming sensitized. Rees *et al.* (1989) used experimental sensitization with DNCB but quantified responses to challenge by measurement of oedema as skin fold thickness. It was shown that, at the particular sensitizing dose used, the proportion of females sensitized was slightly greater, 80 per cent of males cf. 100 per cent of females. However, the females gave much greater responses at each challenge dose and the slope of the dose-response curve was steeper (Rees *et al.*, 1989). This shows that proper quantification can be much more powerful for such comparisons. It also demonstrates that this methodology gives information about both the afferent and efferent components of the immune response, although systemic factors such as heredity, genetics or sex cannot be examined separately on the afferent or efferent limbs of the response. Therefore, in the future, it may be that *in vitro* techniques such as direct enumeration of the numbers of cells specifically sensitized to a particular antigen by limiting dilution analysis will allow sharper analysis of the afferent phase. On the other hand, factors that can be applied locally can be analysed with great discrimination in either the afferent or the local, efferent responses to challenge.

Local Factors in Induction of Contact Sensitivity

As mentioned earlier, systemic factors are likely to affect both afferent and efferent components of the immune response. However, local factors can have an important influence on either the afferent or efferent limbs of the response. As seen from experiments using different sensitizing doses of DNCB, the concentration of antigen is a major determinant of degree of sensitization. In those observations, the concentration of antigen was varied on a fixed area of 3 cm diameter, so in fact the dose per unit area was being changed. The importance of the area itself was explored by changing the area of application and total dose applied while maintaining a constant dose per unit area. As seen from Table 3.1 a total dose of 62.5 μg applied to a 3 cm diameter circle of area 7.1 cm^2 caused clinical sensitivity in only 2 of 24 (8 per cent) subjects. When the same dose of 62.5 μg was applied to a circle 1.5 cm in diameter (1.8 cm^2), 6 of 7 subjects (89 per cent) were sensitized (White *et al.*, 1986a). If the sensitizing stimuli are expressed as concentration per unit area, they are 8.8 and 35.4 μg/cm^2 respectively, a four-fold difference. A dose of 250 μg applied to a 3 cm diameter circle gives a concentration of 35.4 μg/cm^2, i.e., the same as that for 62.5 μg applied to a 1.5 cm circle (Table 3.1). Although the total doses differ by a factor of 4, they have the same sensitizing potency, causing sensitization in 81 per cent of subjects respectively (Table 3.1). Moreover, the degree of reactivity shown

Table 3.1 Relationship between proportions sensitized, area of application, and sensitizing dose of DNCB

Row	Application site Diameter (cm)	Area (cm^2)	Sensitizing dose Total (μg)	Concentration (μg/cm^2)	No. of subjects	Percentage sensitized
1	3	7.1	1000	142	24	100
2	3	7.1	500	71	40	100
3	3	7.1	250	35.4	30	83
4	3	7.1	125	17.7	30	63
5	3	7.1	62.5	8.8	24	8
6	1.5	1.8	62.5	35.4	7	86
7	2.1	3.5	58	16.4	22	55
8	3	7.1	116	16.4	34	50
9	4.25	14.2	232	16.4	15	66
10	1 cm felt	0.8	30	38	28	93
11	3 mm felt	0.08	3	38	15	26

Data from several studies with DNCB. The first 5 rows are the normal subjects from Figures 3.3 and 3.4. Row 6 gives the same dose per unit area as Row 3. In Rows 7–9 the areas were half and double the standard 7.1 cm^2 but the dose per unit area was constant. (Reproduced from Friedmann, 1989a, with permission)

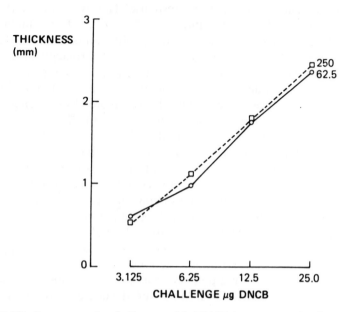

RESPONSES FOR SUBJECTS SENSITISED
WITH SAME CONCENTRATION:
35.4 μg/cm^2

Figure 3.12 Responses to challenge with DNCB in groups of subjects sensitized with the same dose per unit area, 35.4 μg per cm^2 of DNCB. □ = Subjects successfully sensitized with 250 μg on a 3 cm diameter circle, ○ = subjects sensitized with 62.5 μg on a 1.5 cm diameter circle. (Reproduced from White *et al.*, 1986, with permission)

by the sensitized subjects in the two groups was found to be identical (White *et al.*, 1986a) (Figure 3.12). These observations were extended by choosing another concentration – 16.4 μg/cm^2 of DNCB. Three groups were sensitized at this concentration but the area and total dose applied were varied (Table 3.1). Thus, one group received 232 μg on a 4.25 cm circle, one group received 116 μg on a 3 cm diameter circle and one group received 58 μg on a 2.1 cm diameter circle. Again, the proportion sensitized were not significantly different – 55, 50 and 66 per cent respectively ($p<0.5$) (White *et al.*, 1986a). Also, the degree of reactivity elicited by challenge was not significantly different between the three groups (White *et al.*, 1986a). From these results it might be predicted that there would be no reduction of sensitization if the area of application were reduced to an infinitesimal size. To test this prediction a group of people were sensitized using the smallest practicable area. To achieve this 30 μg of DNCB in acetone was applied to a standard 1 cm Al-test disc to give a concentration of 38 μg/cm^2. This stimulus (0.8 cm^2) sensitized 90 per cent of the normal subjects. Discs 3 mm in diameter

$(0.08 \, \text{cm}^2)$ were cut out with a biopsy punch and applied as sensitizing stimulus (Table 3.1). The concentration was still $38 \, \mu\text{g}/\text{cm}^2$ but this area of application was one-tenth that of the 1 cm patch. This induced clinical sensitization in only 26 per cent and their degree of responsiveness was reduced in proportion (Rees *et al.*, 1990).

Overall, these observations indicate that at a given concentration of DNCB per unit area the effect of increasing the area of application, and hence the total dose of DNCB, reaches a plateau above which increases in area cause very little increase in sensitizing effect. Below that plateau, changes in area and total dose exhibit a dose-response relationship as might be expected. These findings can be interpreted in terms of the relationship between the numbers of Langerhans cells and the numbers of antigen molecules per cell. Hence, for a fixed number of Langerhans cells within a given area, varying the number of antigen molecules per cell causes potent changes in the induction stimulus. In contrast, at any given number of molecules per Langerhans cell – constant concentration per unit area – altering the number of antigen-bearing Langerhans cells above a particular plateau level makes only a small difference to sensitivity. Below this plateau, however, changing the number of Langerhans cells has a strong influence on sensitization (Friedmann, 1989b, 1991). This interpretation is supported by the observations of Macatonia *et al.* (1986). They showed that, in mice, increasing the concentration of sensitizing antigen resulted in dose-related increases in the numbers of antigen-bearing Langerhans cells in the regional lymph nodes. Moreover, there was a dose-related increase in the amount of antigen per Langerhans cell.

Local Factors in Expression of Contact Sensitivity

Anatomical site significantly affects cutaneous inflammatory reactivity. This has been demonstrated most clearly with irritant substances. Thus, reactivity to the irritant dimethylsulphoxide (DMSO) is greatest on the forehead with progressively reduced reactivity on the upper back, ante-cubital fossa, forearm, lower leg and wrist (Vandervalk and Maibach, 1989; Frosch, 1992). Similar variations were found in response to benzalkonium chloride (Magnusson and Hersle, 1965), and Lawrence *et al.* (1986) showed with anthralin, another irritant, that responses on the forearm exhibited consistent site-related variations, responsiveness was greater proximally and laterally.

Local factors are also important in the expression of immune responses in skin and these will have an important effect on the clinical manifestations of contact sensitivity as well as the responses to formal challenge. Magnusson and Hersle (1965) performed simultaneous patch tests on several body sites of people known to be sensitized to the test antigen. Upper back was most reactive, followed by lower back, forearm, upper arm and thigh. In the account of normal responses to DNCB above, it was argued that the slope of dose-response curves for response measured as change of skin thickness reflected local cutaneous inflammatory factors. This also appears to apply for the slope of the dose-response curve when measured as erythema with a reflectance instrument. The experimental confirmation of this was obtained by quantification of responses to serial dilutions of nickel patients (Memon and Friedmann, unpublished data). Four-fold dilutions of nickel sulphate from 5 per cent downwards, were applied on Finn chambers for 48 hours. The responses were graded clinically as "positive" when there was palpable erythema, and quantified with a reflectance instrument by measurement of increase in erythema over base-line. The back was much more reactive in that the threshold concentration required to produce a positive response was one-quarter to one-eighth of the threshold on the forearm. Also, the slope of the erythema dose-response curve was much steeper (Memon and Friedmann, unpublished data). These local differences in reactivity may result in clinical problems from certain substances such as cosmetics occurring on one area, for instance the face, but not on other areas such as the hands.

Potentiation of Allergic Responses

A clinical problem that arises is seen when a person appears to become allergic to something such as a cosmetic, but patch test challenge with the separate ingredients applied in the standard concentrations fails to detect the contact sensitivity. This apparent methodological weakness of patch testing can be explained by results from an interesting study by McLelland and Shuster (1990). Since allergic contact hypersensitivity responses are dose-related, it is clear that doubling the concentration of an antigen will increase the strength of the response. If the concentration of antigen is below the threshold level, then if doubled, it may come above the threshold and so elicit a "positive" response. McLelland showed this in people who were sensitive to two different contact allergens. They were challenged with a doubling dilution series of each antigen separately and also combined at each dilution. There was a complete summation so that at any concentration, the response to the two antigens combined was about the same as the sum of the individual responses at that concentration. Moreover, mixtures of antigens at sub-clinical levels indeed crossed the threshold and elicited clinically detectable responses (McLelland and Shuster, 1990).

A similar phenomenon was shown when an irritant was substituted for one of the antigens (McLelland *et al.*, 1991). The method was slightly different, but when sites challenged with a sub-threshold dose of antigen for 24 hours were given the additional irritant challenge for the second 24 hours, then significant clinically positive responses were obtained. A similar but less well quantified study was performed by Sonnex and Ryan (1987). They showed that pretreatment of skin with Thurfyl nicotinate cream, a rubefacient, followed by patch testing with 20 substances causes a significant increase in the number of positive patch test reactions.

It is clear that an irritant may augment absorption of antigen, raising its effective concentration. Also, as will be seen below, irritants like antigens activate processes in the skin aimed at recruitment of immune surveillance mechanisms. The two stimuli for these mechanisms can clearly summate to increase the likelihood of antigen specific effector T cells entering the tissues to encounter the low dose of antigen.

"Angry Back" and "Excited Skin Syndrome"

These terms must be mentioned because they are often alluded to in the clinical practice of diagnostic patch testing. The term "angry back" was coined by Mitchell in relation to the phenomenon of multiple positive patch test reactions occurring on the same individual (Mitchell and Maibach, 1982). He showed that if substances giving weak (+) reactions were retested singly at a later time, a significant proportion (42 per cent) were negative. He presumed this meant they were, in fact, false positive and did not represent genuine sensitization. Bruynzeel performed a similar study and arrived at a similar conclusion (Brunyzeel *et al.*, 1983b). By contrast, Bandman and Agathos (1981) found only 8.6 per cent of such so-called false positive responses became negative upon retesting. The difference has been explained on the basis of different methodology, including retesting strong reactions as well as weak ones. Maibach broadened the term to "excited skin syndrome" to indicate that a generalized hyper-irritability could occur in skin (Maibach, 1981). The central tenet of the idea is that one strong patch test reaction creates the hyper-reactive state. Evidence that this is not so was presented by Kligman and Gollhausen (1986). They first challenged a range of volunteers with irritants or sensitizers to which they were sensitive, to obtain base-line responses. Then, they generated strong responses with sensitizers such as DNCB, nickel or rhus oleoresin of poison ivy. They placed the challenges at the corners of a square on the backs of subjects sensitized to these agents. Then, various challenges with either irritants or sensitizers were placed within the squares. No augmentation was seen of any response compared with the base line. The present author has made similar but less comprehensive observations (unpublished data). This would seem to cast serious doubt on the concept that a general phenomenon exists in which a strong local patch test or irritant response can induce hyper-reactivity. However, Magnusson and Helgren (1962) observed that when test subjects developed a reaction due to the adhesive tape used to apply patch tests, a much greater frequency of positive responses was seen. Also, Brunyzeel *et al.* (1983a) showed that guinea pigs pre-treated with Freund's complete adjuvant became hyper-reactive both to allergens and irritants. These two observations add the perspective which is, in fact, present in slightly loose form in the literature, that hyper-irritability is seen when there is active dermatitis present.

There is still much work to be done to define the conditions under which such hyper-reactivity occurs. However, it is conceivable that the prerequisite is for the presence of active skin inflammation that is accompanied by increased levels of circulating cytokines. These could have the effect of priming the skin vasculature in the same way a local, sub-threshold applications of irritant or allergen – as seen with Trafuril pretreatment performed by Sonnex and Ryan (1987). The question that preoccupies clinicians of whether reactions on an angry back are genuine or false positive may be resolved by *in vitro* techniques such as analysis of the antigenic specificities of reacting lymphocytes.

Recruitment of Immune Surveillance Mechanisms in Skin

As mentioned in the introduction to this chapter, a vital function of skin is in defence against invasion by microbes. Since the skin is under continuous assault by chemical substances in the environment, it seems probable that efficient mechanisms must be present to activate or recruit immune surveillance to "inspect" any substance that penetrates from outside. The critical event in a cell-mediated immune response to an antigen is the specific interaction between the antigen, presented in association with MHC class II determinants, on the surface of an antigen presenting cell and the relevant T cell receptor on the surface of a $CD4^+$ T lymphocyte. After this interaction the T cell responds by releasing cytokines of which interferon-γ (IFN-γ) appears most important, to augment the recruitment of other lympho-mononuclear cells (Issekutz *et al.*, 1988). When an antigen enters the skin, the statistical likelihood is very low of a chance encounter between the antigen and a specifically committed T cell trafficking through the tissues. This jeopardizes the protective efficiency of immune surveillance and it is becoming clear that the skin plays an active role in increasing the efficiency of the response.

It could be predicted that chemical or even physical perturbation would activate mechanisms to increase trafficking of T cells through the tissues. Furthermore, such recruitment mechanisms must be non-specific in that they cannot distinguish whether or not the provoking substance is microbial in origin. Moreover, these mechanisms must operate independently of whether or not the host has been previously sensitized and in addition they must become activated rapidly.

A number of studies have found evidence of these mechanisms by examining skin after application of various chemical provoking substances including irritants and "antigens" to which mice (Malorny *et al.*, 1988) or humans were known to be specifically "sensitive" or "non-sensitive" (Griffiths and Nickoloff, 1989; Griffiths *et al.*, 1991; Sterry *et al.*, 1991; Friedmann *et al.*, 1993). The main changes detected relate on the one hand to increased numbers of putative antigen presenting cells in the superficial dermis, and on the other hand to changes in expression of cell adhesion molecules on dermal microvascular endothelium and, also in some circumstances, on epidermal keratinocytes.

In pre-challenge resting skin some dermal vessels express intercellular adhesion molecule 1 (ICAM-1) but generally endothelial cell leucocyte adhesion molecule 1 (ELAM-1) and vascular cell adhesion molecule 1 (VCAM-1) are not detectable. The scanty population of immune cells is mainly perivascular and comprises $CD3^+$ T cells, $CD14^+$ macrophages and occasional $CD1a^+$ Langerhans cells. In the epidermis, although $CD1a^+$ Langerhans cells are present, there is no expression of ICAM-1 and, depending on the antibody used, some staining of basal cells for tumour necrosis factor-α (TNF-α) and interleukin-1α (IL-1α) can be detected (Friedmann *et al.*, 1993). After challenge with irritants or sensitizers such as nickel, *p*-phenylenediamine, urushiol or DNCB, and regardless of whether individuals are "sensitive" or not, there are similar changes seen up to 8 hours.

Immune Cells

By 2–4 hours after challenge there is an increase in the numbers of $CD1a^+$ Langerhans cells in the superficial dermis. This change appears proportional to the "strength" of the provoking agent, occurring most with irritants such as anthralin, or highly potent sensitizers such as DNCB (Friedmann *et al.*, 1993). However, it is even seen at 24 hours with innocuous chemical mixtures such as white soft paraffin (Sterry *et al.*, 1991). No changes are detected in the dermal mononuclear cell infiltrate up to 8 hours. However, by 24 hours skin biopsies from subjects "sensitized" to the provoking substances show a significant mononuclear cell infiltrate comprised mainly of T cells of phenotype $CD3^+$, $CD4^+$, $CD45RO^+$, which represent memory T cells. Among the T cells, occasional cells were observed that expressed CD25, the p55 chain of the IL-2 receptor. This marker is thought to be expressed by T cells that have been activated following binding of the T cell receptor with its homologous antigen/MHC-class II complex (Meuer *et al.*, 1984). A few $CD4^+$ T cells are seen in the epidermis, while deeper in the dermis $CD14^+$ monocyte/macrophages are increased. In sensitized individuals generating "positive" responses to antigen challenge, the T cell infiltrate continues to increase to 48 hours at which time many $CD1b^+$ dermal dendrocytes are seen adjacent to superficial dermal capillaries. Interestingly, these cells are strongly stained by anti-VCAM-1 antibodies (Friedmann *et al.*, 1993). In the fully developed reaction, IL-8 expression is seen on keratinocytes too (Griffiths *et al.*, 1991).

Changes in Adhesion Molecules

Increased expression in ICAM-1, ELAM-1 and VCAM-1 was first detectable after only 2 hours and increased in intensity to reach a maximum at 24 hours

(Figure 3.13). Interestingly, in people known to be sensitive to the challenge substance, and also at sites challenged with irritants, the numbers of vessels expressing ICAM-1 also showed a significant increase at 8 hours (Figure 3.14) (Friedmann *et al.*, 1993). Some authors have also found that ICAM-1 is expressed in focal patches on basal keratinocytes. Griffiths *et al.* (1989, 1991) found this at 4 hours with progressive increase with time, while others have found it only by 24 hours after challenge (Sterry *et al.*, 1991).

In summary, these observations appear to indicate the following sequence of events following chemical perturbation. There is a rapid (2 hours) increase in numbers of dermal Langerhans cells which have been shown to carry antigens (Carr *et al.*, 1984). Also, rapid upregulation in expression of adhesion molecules by dermal microvascular endothelium is seen. This appears to be a direct effect since it is seen with cultured endothelial cells too (Meinardus-Hager *et al.*, 1992). There may also be expression of ICAM-1 by keratinocytes, although this is not detected by most workers. Moreover, keratinocytes exposed to urushiol *in vitro* express ICAM-1 by 48 hours (Griffiths and Nickoloff, 1989; Barker *et al.*, 1991). Thus, the conditions are established to recruit T cells to perform immune surveillance. Activated memory T cells are particularly rich in lymphocyte function associated antigen-1 (LFA-1) and cutaneous lymphocyte antigen (CLA), the ligands for ICAM-1 and ELAM-1 respectively (Berg *et al.*, 1991; Picker *et al.*, 1991; Shimizu *et al.*, 1991). Therefore, the initial expression of ELAM-1 and ICAM-1 by endothelial cells is probably sufficient to allow attachment of T cells to the endothelium. After attachment, the T cells must express β1-integrins including VLA-3, 5 and 6 which are ligands for collagen, fibronectin and laminin, which will be required for emigration into the tissues (Butcher, 1991). If no T cell recognizes its target antigen, the whole reaction subsides over a few hours. However, once a specifically committed T cell recognizes its target antigen on the surface of a Langerhans cell, it becomes activated, expressing CD25 and releasing cytokines including IFN-γ and TNF-α. These will upregulate adhesion molecule expression further and recruit other T cells into the area to participate in the inflammatory reaction clinically as allergic contact eczema.

These observations made in humans demonstrate no qualitative differences between the early effects of substances that are sensitizers or irritants, while the distinctive consequences of activation of sensitized T cells only develop from 8 hours at the earliest. Similar findings were made in mice by Malorny *et al.* (1988). However, a study by Enk and Katz (1992) used sensitive molecular biological techniques to detect mRNA for various cytokines after mice were treated with irritant (sodium lauryl sulphate), haptens and also tolerogens. They observed certain differences in early, 4-hour, profiles of cytokines. Although TNF-α, IFN-γ and granulocyte/macrophage colony-stimulating factor (GM-CSF) were increased in the epidermis by all compounds, only the contact sensitizers upregulated IL-1α, IL-1β, MHC Class II and macrophage inflammatory protein 2(MIP-2). It remains to be

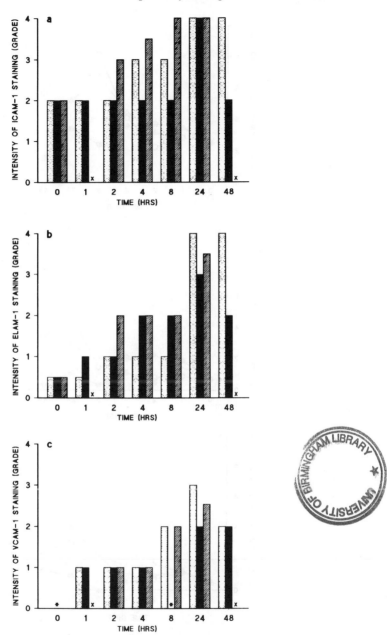

Figure 3.13 Intensity of staining of adhesion molecules at various times after challenge. ▨ = Reaction in individuals known to be sensitive to the challenge, ■ = reaction in individuals known to be non-sensitized to the challenge, □ = irritant reactions. Panels a) ICAM-1, b) ELAM-1, c) VCAM-1. * = No staining observed; X = no biopsies at these time points. (Reproduced from Friedmann *et al.*, 1993, with permission)

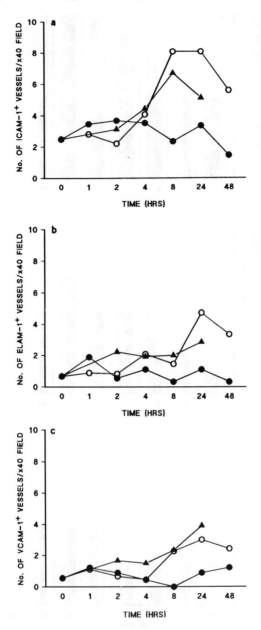

Figure 3.14 Adhesion molecule expression by dermal microvascular endothelial cells at various times after epicutaneous challenge. ○ = Reaction in individuals known to be sensitive to provoking stimulus, ● = reaction in subjects known to be non-sensitive to provoking stimulus, ▲ = irritant reactions. Panels a) ICAM-1, b) ELAM-1, c) VCAM-1. Points are numbers of vessels per 40× high power field. (Reproduced from Friedmann *et al.*, 1993, with permission)

seen whether human skin will also show these qualitative differences in response to exposure to different types of provoking chemical.

Conclusions

In conclusion, studies of the clinical response of allergic contact dermatitis have led to a greatly increased understanding of the behaviour of the immune system, the recognition that independent of the immune status of the host, the skin can "sense" physical or chemical perturbation. This results in activation of a complex response, from which explanation of many phenomena observed clinically becomes possible. For instance, it shows why sub-threshold concentrations of antigens and/or irritants can summate to generate clinically detectable responses. If the non-specific recruitment mechanisms are activated to a greater extent, the chance of an antigen specific T cell entering the tissues to find its antigen will be increased in proportion. Also, it becomes apparent that repeated exposure to irritant chemicals with chronic activation of these mechanisms including adhesion molecules and cytokines, aimed at recruiting the "machinery" of immune surveillance, can indeed generate a non-specific inflammatory or "irritant" reaction.

References

AGRUP, G. (1969) Hand eczema and other dermatoses in South Sweden. *Acta Dermatol. Vener.* (Suppl.), **49**, 61.

BANDMAN, H-J. and AGATHOS, M. (1981) New results and some remarks to the "angry back syndrome". *Contact Dermatitis*, **7**, 23–6.

BARKER, J.N., MITRA, R.S., GRIFFITHS, C.E., DIXIT, V.M., and NICKOLOFF, B.J. (1991) Keratinocytes as initiators of inflammation. *Lancet*, **337**, 211–14.

BERG, E.L., YOSHINO, T., ROTT, L.S., ROBINSON, M.K., WARNOCK, R.A., KISHIMOTO, T.K., PICKER, L.J., and BUTCHER, E.C. (1991) The cutaneous lymphocyte antigen is a skin lymphocyte homing receptor for the vascular lectin endothelial cell-leukocyte adhesion molecule 1. *J. Exp. Med.*, **174**, 1461–6.

BLEUMINK, E., NATER, J.P., KOOPS, S., and THE, T.H. (1974) A standard method for DNCB sensitization testing in patients with neoplasms. *Cancer*, **33**, 911–15.

BRUNYZEEL, D.P., VAN KETEL, W.G., VON BLOMBERK-VAN DER FLIER, B.M.E., and SCHEPER, R.J. (1983a) Angry back or the excited skin syndrome. *J. Am. Acad. Dermatol.*, **8**, 392–7.

BRUNYZEEL, D.P., VON BLOMBERG-VAN DER FLIER, B.M.E, VAN KETEL, W.G., et al. (1983b) Depression or enhancement of skin reactivity by inflammatory processes in the guinea pig. *Int. Arch. Allergy Appl. Immunol.*, **72**, 67–70.

BUTCHER, E.C. (1991) Leucocyte-endothelial cell recognition: three (or more) steps to specificity and diversity. *Cell*, **67**, 1033–36.

CARR, M.M., BOTHAM, P.A., GAWKROGER, D.J., McVITTIE, E.M., ROSS, J.A., STEWART, I.C., and HUNTER, J.A.A. (1984) Early cellular reactions induced by dinitrochlorbenzene in sensitized human skin. *Brit. J. Dermatol.*, **110**, 637–41.

CATALONA, W.J., TAYLOR, P.Y., RABSON, A.S., and CHRETIEN, P.B. (1972) A method for dinitrochlorobenzene contact sensitization. *New Eng. J. Med*, **286**, 362–7.

DE BERKER, D., IBBOTSON, S., SIMPSON, N.B., MATTHEWS, J.N.S, IDLE, J.R., and REES, J.L. (1995) Reduced experimental contact sensitivity in squamous cell but not basal cell carcinomas of the skin. *Lancet*, **345**, 425–6.

EILBER, F.R. and MORTON, D.L. (1970) Impaired immunologic reactivity and recurrence following cancer surgery. *Cancer*, **25**, 362–7.

EMMET, E.A. (1984) The skin and occupational disease. *Arch. Environ. Health*, **39**, 144–9.

ENK, A.H. and KATZ, S.I. (1992) Early molecular events in the induction phase of contact sensitivity. *Proc. Natl. Acad. Sci. USA*, **89**, 1398–402.

EPSTEIN, W.L. and MAIBACH, H.I. (1965) Immunologic compentence of patients with psoriasis receiving cytotoxic drug therapy. *Arch. Dermatol.*, **91**, 599–606.

FRIEDMANN, P.S., MOSS, C., SHUSTER, S., and SIMPSON, J.M. (1983) Quantitative relationships between sensitizing dose of DNCB and reactivity in normal subjects. *Clin. Exp. Immunol.*, **53**, 709–11.

FRIEDMANN, P.S. (1986) Immune functions of skin. In: Scientific basis of dermatology. A physiological approach. A.J. Thody and P.S. Friedmann (eds), Churchill Livingstone, Edinburgh, pp. 58–73.

(1989a) The immunology of allergic contact dermatitis: The DNCB story. In: Advances in Dermatology. M.V. Dahl (ed.), Year Book Medical Publishers, Chicago, Illinois, Vol. 5, pp. 175–95.

(1989b) Contact hypersensitivity. *Curr. Opin. Immunol.*, **1**, 690–3.

(1991) Graded continuity, or all or none – studies of the human immune response. *Clin. Exp. Dermatol.*, **16**, 79–84.

FRIEDMANN, P.S., REES, J., WHITE, S.I., and MATTHEWS, J.N. (1990) Low-dose exposure to antigen induces sub-clinical sensitization. *Clin. Exp. Immunol.*, **81**, 507–9.

FRIEDMANN, P.S., STRICKLAND, I., MEMON, A.A., and JOHNSON, P.M. (1993) Early time course of recruitment of immune surveillance in human skin after chemical provocation. *Clin. Exp. Immunol.*, **91**, 351–6.

FRIEDMANN, P.S. and MOSS, C. (1985) Quantification of contact hypersensitivity in man. In: Models in Dermatology. H.I. Maibach and N.J. Lowe (eds), Karger, Basle, pp. 275–81.

FROSCH, P.J. (1992) Cutaneous irritation. In: Textbook of contact dermatitis. R.J.G. Rycroft, T. Menne, P.J. Frosch and C. Benezra (eds), Springer-Verlag, Berlin, pp. 28–60.

GRIFFITHS, C.E.M., BARKER, J.N.W.N., KUNKEL, S., and NICKOLOFF, B.J. (1991) Modulation of leucocyte adhesion molecules, a T-cell chemotaxin (IL-8) and a regulatory cytokine (TNF-a) in allergic contact dermatitis (rhus dermatitis). *Brit. J. Dermatol.*, **124**, 519–26.

GRIFFITHS, C.E.M. and NICKOLOFF, B.J. (1989) Keratinocyte adhesion molecule-1 (ICAM-1) expression precedes dermal T lymphocyte infiltration in allergic contact dermatitis (rhus dermatitis). *Am. J. Pathol.*, **135**, 1045–53.

ISSEKUTZ, T.B., STOLTZ, J.M., and VAN DER MEIDE, P. (1988) Lymphocyte recruitment in delayed-type hypersensitivity: the role of IFN-γ. *J. Immunol.*, **140**, 2989–93.

JORDAN, J.L. and KING, S.E. (1977) Delayed hypersensitivity in females. *Contact Dermatitis*, **3**, 19–26.

JOHNSON, M.L.T. and ROBERTS, J. (1978) Skin conditions and related need for medical care among persons 1–74 years. *Vital Health Stat.*, **11**.

KAVLI, G. and FORDE, O.H. (1984) Hand dermatoses in Tromso. *Contact Dermatitis*, **10**, 174–7.

KINNAIRD, A., PETERS, S.W., FOSTER, J.R., and KIMBER, I. (1989) Dendritic cell accumulation in draining lymph nodes during the induction phase of contact allergy in mice. *Int. Arch. Allergy Appl. Immunol.*, **89**, 202–10.

KLIGMAN, A. and GOLLHAUSEN, R. (1986) The "angry back": a new concept or old confusion? *Brit. J. Dermatol.*, **115** suppl., 93–100.

LEYDEN, J.J. and KLIGMAN, A.M. (1977) Allergic contact dermatitis: sex differences. *Contact Dermatitis*, **3**, 333–6.

MACATONIA, S.E., EDWARDS, A.J., and KNIGHT, S.C. (1986) Dendritic cells and the initiation of contact sensitivity to fluorescein isothiocyanate. *Immunol.*, **59**, 509–14.

MAGNUSSON, B. and HELGREN, L. (1962) Skin irritating and adhesive characteristics of some different tapes. *Acta Derm. Venereol.*, **42**, 463–72.

MAGNUSSON, B. and HERSLE, K. (1965) Patch test methods II: regional variations of patch test responses. *Acta Derm. Venereol.*, **45**, 257–61.

MAIBACH, H.I. (1981) The ESS: excited skin syndrome. In: New trends in allergy. J. Ring and G. Burg (eds), Springer-Verlag, New York, pp. 208–21.

MALORNY, U., KNOP, J., BURMEISTER, G., and SORG, C. (1988) Immunohistochemical demonstration of migration inhibitory factor (MIF) in experimental allergic contact dermatitis. *Clin. Exp. Immunol.*, **71**, 164–70.

MATHIAS, C.G.T. (1985) The cost of occupational disease. *Arch. Dermatol.*, **121**, 332–4.

McLELLAND, J., SHUSTER, S., and MATTHEWS, J.N. (1991) 'Irritants' increase the response to an allergen in allergic contact dermatitis. *Arch. Dermatol.*, **127**, 1016–19.

MEDING, B.E. and SWANBECK, G. (1987) Prevalence of hand eczema in an industrial city. *Brit. J. Dermatol.*, **116**, 627–34.

MEINARDUS-HAGER, G., GOEBELER, M., GUTWALD, J., and SORG, C. (1992) The allergen nickel chloride directly induces distinct expression patterns of leucocyte adhesion molecules on human endothelial cells. *J. Invest. Dermatol.*, **98**, 539.

MENNE, T. and HOLM, N.V. (1983) Hand eczema in nickel-sensitive female twins. *Contact Dermatitis*, **9**, 289–96.

(1986) Genetic susceptibility in human allergic contact sensitization. *Semin. Dermatol.*, **5**, 301–6.

MEUER, S.C., HUSSEY, R.E., CANTRELL, D., HODGDON, J.C., SCHLOSSMAN, S.F., SMITH, K.A., and REINHERZ, E.L. (1984) Triggering of the T3-Ti antigen receptor complex results in clonal T-cell proliferation through an interleukin-2 dependent autocrine pathway. *Proc. Natl. Acad. Sci. USA*, **81**, 1509–13.

MITCHELL, J.C. and MAIBACH, H.I. (1982) The angry back syndrome: the excited skin syndrome. *Seminars in Dermatol.*, **1**, 9–13.

MOSS, C. (1983) Studies of cutaneous sensitization to dinitrochlorobenzene in man.

MD Thesis, Oxford University.

MOSS, C., FRIEDMANN, P.S., SHUSTER, S., and SIMPSON, J.M. (1985) Susceptibility and amplification of sensitivity in contact dermatitis. *Clin. Exp. Immunol.*, **61**, 232–41.

OKAMOTO, K. and KRIKE, M.L. (1987) Effector and suppressor circuits of the immune response are activated *in vivo* by different mechanisms. *Proc. Natl. Acad. Sci. USA*, **84**, 3841–5.

PICKER, L.J., KISHIMOTO, T.K., SMITH, C.W., WARNOCK, R.A., and BUTCHER, E.C. (1991) ELAM-1 is an adhesion molecule for skin-homing T cells. *Nature*, **349**, 796–9.

POLAK, L., BARNES, J.M., and TURK, J.L. (1968) The genetic control of contact sensitization to inorganic metal compounds in guinea pigs. *Immunology*, **14**, 707–11.

REA, J.N., NEWHOUSE, M.L., and HALIL, T. (1976) Skin diseases in Lambeth. A community study of prevalence and use of medical care. *Brit. J. Prev. Soc. Med.*, **30**, 107–14.

REES, J.L., FRIEDMANN, P.S., and MATTHEWS, J.N.S. (1989) Sex differences in susceptibility to development of contact hypersensitivity to dinitrochlorobenzene. *Brit. J. Dermatol.*, **120**, 371–4.

REES, J.L., FRIEDMANN, P.S., and MATTHEWS, J.N. (1990) The influence of area of application on sensitization by dinitrochlorobenzene. *Brit. J. Dermatol.*, **122**, 29–31.

ROSTENBERG, A. and KANOFF, N.M. (1941) Studies in eczematous sensitizations. *J. Invest. Dermatol.*, **4**, 505–13.

SCHWARTZ, M. (1953) Eczematous sensitization in various age groups. *J. Allergy*, **24**, 143–8.

SHIMIZU, Y., SHAW, S., GRABER, N., GOPAL, T.V., HORGAN, K.J., VAN SEVENTER, G.A., and NEWMAN, W. (1991) Activation-independent binding of human memory T cells to adhesion molecule ELAM-1. *Nature*, **349**, 799–802.

SONNEX, T.S. and RYAN, T.J (1987) An investigation of the angry back syndrome using Trafuril. *Brit. J. Dermatol.*, **116**, 361–70.

STERRY, W., KUNNE, N., WEBER-MATTHIESEN, K., BRASCH, J., and MIELKE, V. (1991) Cell trafficking in positive and negative patch-test reactions: Demonstration of a stereotypic migration pathway. *J. Invest. Dermatol.*, **96**, 459–62.

VANDERVALK, P.G.M. and MAIBACH, H.I. (1989) Potential for irritation increases from the wrist to the cubital fossa. *Brit. J. Dermatol.*, **121**, 709–12.

WALKER, F.B., SMITH, P.O., and MAIBACH, H.I. (1967) Genetic factors in human allergic contact dermatitis. *Int. Arch. Allergy Appl. Immunol.*, **32**, 453–62.

WHITE, S.I., FRIEDMANN, P.S., MOSS, C., and SIMPSON, J.M. (1986a) The effect of altering area of application and dose per unit area on sensitization by DNCB. *Brit. J. Dermatol.*, **115**, 663–8.

WHITE, S.I., FRIEDMANN, P.S., and STRATTON, A. (1986b) HLA antigens and Langerhans' cell density in contact dermatitis. *Brit. J. Dermatol.*, **115**, 447–52.

4

Occupational Allergic Contact Dermatitis

J.E. WAHLBERG

Karolinska Hospital, Stockholm

Occupational Dermatoses

Occupational dermatoses such as irritant and allergic contact dermatitis, contact urticaria, oil- and chloracne, hyper- and hypopigmentation, chemical burns and squamous cell carcinoma are caused mainly by chemicals and chemical products. Other causes are radiation, friction (mechanical trauma), infections (bacteria, virus, fungi).

Depending on the country, dermatoses comprise from 20 to 70 per cent of all occupational disease, and between 20 and 90 per cent of these are contact dermatitis. Irritant contact dermatitis is considered to be more prevalent than allergic, partly as a result of more extensive and precise preventive measures including predictive testing. The proportion of allergic contact dermatitis to irritant contact dermatitis is determined by the extent and type of industrialization in an area, and by the skill, interest and commitment of dermatologists regarding contact dermatitis – its causes, diagnosis, treatment and prevention.

In a paper by Griffiths (1985), 'Industrial dermatitis – a national problem', the issue is discussed in greater detail. The cost implications of occupational dermatoses are reviewed by Mathias (1985).

Definition of Occupational Contact Dermatitis

There is no universally accepted definition of occupational contact dermatitis (Rycroft, 1995). A common definition is contact dermatitis due wholly or partially to the patient's occupation. According to stricter definition occupational exposure should be the major factor. An alternative definition is contact dermatitis that would not have occurred if the worker had not been exposed at work. The medicolegal aspects vary from country to country (Frosch and Rycroft, 1995).

Contact Allergens

There are 3700 chemicals described that can cause allergic contact dermatitis (de Groot, 1994), and data on new ones are published every year. In de Groot's first book (1986), 2800 allergens were reviewed, indicating that 900 additional chemicals were identified as sensitizers between 1986 and 1994.

Exposure can take place in the work environment as well as at home or in leisure time and there is a considerable overlap. Contact allergy to some plastics, intermediates in chemical synthesis and precursors of drugs in the pharmaceutical industry are clearly work-related, but what about fragrances, mascaras, spices, plants, dental materials? To give an example, contact allergy to fragrances can be contracted by beauticians, cosmetologists, hairdressers and cleaners and to plants by gardeners and florists in their profession.

When examining the individual patient it is sometimes hard to decide whether exposure – at work or in leisure time – is the major cause. Clinically, a primary occupational contact allergy will cause problems and risks of relapses even if the exposure at work has entirely ceased, since the allergens (e.g. nickel, rubber chemicals, preservatives) are abundant also in the non-work environment (see Prognosis).

The opposite situation is common also: the allergy is acquired in private life and a relapse of dermatitis takes place from occupational exposure. An example often quoted is dermatitis of the hands from job contact with nickel (tools etc.) in patients sensitized by nickel in jewellery.

Symptoms and Clinical Picture

Symptoms and Reasons for Seeking Medical Advice

The main symptom is itching which not infrequently will disturb sleep. Patients are afraid of the lesions also appearing in other skin sites, of the risk of communication to workmates and relatives, of the unpleasant or disgusting appearance of the dermatitis or of a dispute with the employer.

Morphology

There is usually a mixture of erythema, oedema, papules, vesicles, pustules, scaling, fissuring and oozing with variation from site to site. In the acute phase of a contact eczema erythema, oedema and oozing may dominate while in more chronic cases scaling, dryness and fissuring are more prominent characteristics.

Distribution

The primary sites of an occupational allergic contact dermatitis are usually the hands, the forearms and the face, but later spreading to other skin sites is not unusual. The location can give some hints as to the inducing agent: chemicals, products, and materials in contact with and contaminating the hands; airborne allergens (e.g. in dusts) to the face and lower legs; protective shoes or boots used at work etc.

Work Relation, Course

A typical case of work-related contact dermatitis will gradually clear when the patient is on sick leave, on vacation etc. and recur when he/she is back at work. However, several contact allergens are so ubiquitous that many patients will not clear even if they are out of work.

Factors Influencing Sensitization

Factors influencing sensitization are summarized in Table 4.1. However, their relative importance is hard to decide. Our well-established knowledge of the allergens originates from clinical experience and from experimental sensitization studies: human maximization testing (Kligman, 1966), 'Modified Draize' (Marzulli and Maibach, 1973) and human repeat insult patch test (Griffith and Buehler, 1977), while our knowledge of host and environmental factors is scantier. It is challenging that we still do not know why some of those exposed to an allergen at work become sensitized while the majority appear to be resistant. We would like deeper knowledge of genetic factors, how they interplay with the allergens and how they thereby influence sensitization and the development of tolerance.

Diagnostic Procedures

Patch Testing

Patch testing, introduced in 1895 (Jadassohn), is a well-established *in vivo* method of diagnosing allergic contact dermatitis. Patients with a history of suspected exposure to allergens, and a clinical picture of contact dermatitis

Table 4.1 Factors influencing contact allergic sensitization in humans

Allergen	Physicochemical properties
	Sensitizing potential
	Concentration, dose
	Nature of vehicle
	Frequency of exposure
	Exposure under occlusion
Host	Skin site
	Density of Langerhans' cells
	Pre-existing irritant dermatitis
	Pre-existing skin barrier defect
	Genetic predisposition
	Age
	Sex
Environment	Humidity
	Temperature
	Related seasonal factors

Table 4.2 Allergic contact hand eczema

Irritant contact dematitis
Atopic hand eczema
Nummular eczema
Dyshidrotic eczema (pompholyx)
Tylotic eczema
Psoriasis of the hands
Pustulosis palmaris
Photo contact dermatitis
Mycotic infections
Porphyria cutanea tarda
Scabies
Secondary syphilis
Self-inflicted skin lesions (artifacts)

Some differential diagnoses encountered at a Department of Occupational Dermatology.

are re-exposed (under occlusion) to standard allergens and products from the work and leisure environment under controlled conditions to verify the clinical diagnosis. With other types of eczema, too, patch testing is sometimes indicated to permit a differential diagnosis (Table 4.2), or when the dermatologist suspects contact allergy to prescribed topical medicaments.

Besides its use to confirm a suspected diagnosis of allergic contact dermatitis, patch testing can be used also when looking for alternatives to an allergen-containing product. If particular patients do not react to the

Table 4.3   European standard patch test series

---

1. Potassium dichromate
2. 4-Phenylenediamine base
3. Thiuram mix (4 rubber chemicals)
4. Neomycin sulphate
5. Cobalt chloride
6. Benzocaine
7. Nickel sulphate
8. Clioquinol
9. Colophony
10. Paraben mix (4 esters, preservatives)
11. N-Isopropyl-N-phenyl-4-phenylenediamine (antidegradant)
12. Wool alcohols
13. Mercapto mix (4 rubber chemicals)
14. Epoxy resin
15. Balsam of Peru
16. 4-tert-Butylphenol formaldehyde resin
17. Mercaptobenzothiazole (rubber chemical)
18. Formaldehyde
19. Fragrance mix (8 fragrances)
20. Sesquitererpene lactone mix (3 plant allergens)
21. Quaternium 15 (preservative)
22. Primin
23. Cl + Me isothiazolinone (preservative)

Chemotechnique, 1994/95; Hermal, 1994.

alternatives tested (e.g. glove materials, skin care products), it is very unlikely that they will react to the products in ordinary use. The patch test method is today considered to be accurate and reliable since much effort has been put into standardization of allergens, vehicles, concentrations, materials such as patches and tapes, and into the system for scoring test reactions.

Test Procedure

For details the reader is referred to current textbooks (Adams and Fischer, 1990; Fisher, 1986; Wahlberg, 1995).

Test systems: Two test systems can be distinguished: the original one, where the allergens, patches and tapes are supplied separately, and the modern ready-to-use method (i.e. TRUE-test), where only a covering material has to be removed before the test is applied.

Patches: In the original system there are at least three types in current use: Al-test, Finn chambers and van der Bend test patches.

Allergens: Two suppliers, Hermal (1994) and Chemotechnique (1994/95), offer more than 300 contact allergens, and their annual catalogues contain details of formulas, synonyms, vehicles, concentrations, presence in products and the environment and cross reactivity. In Table 4.3 the present standard test series is shown, as recommended by the European Environmental and Contact Dermatitis Research Group (EECDRG). Among the standard allergens and mixes of allergens, the majority are relevant for occupational exposure.

Test site: The upper back is recommended.

Exposure time: 2 days (48 hours).

Reading time: Two readings are recommended, one at 48 hours after removal of patches and a second 2–4 days later.

Recording of test reactions: The presence of erythema, oedema, papules, vesicles and bullae is recorded and quantified.

Interpretation: To distinguish allergic reactions from irritant reactions on morphological grounds only is difficult. Weak reactions especially – erythema with or without infiltration – are controversial in interpretation. In these cases repeat tests, increased concentrations, serial dilution tests and repeated open application tests (ROATs, see below) are recommended.

Relevance: Evaluating the relevance of a positive patch test reaction is the most difficult part of the procedure. The dermatologist's experience, skill and curiosity are important factors for the outcome.

For the standard allergens detailed lists provide information on the occurrence of each allergen in the environment (Table 4.3). These lists should be studied together by patient and dermatologist. The relevance of a positive patch test reaction in relation to exposure, affected skin site(s), course and reported relapses can then be evaluated. It sometimes remains unexplained until a tube, a bottle, a container etc., where the allergen in question is named on the label, is brought by the patient. In other cases, chemical analyses will demonstrate the presence of a particular allergen (see below).

For discussions of cross reactivity, false-positive and false-negative test reactions, effects of medicaments and irradiation on patch test reactions, complications, for example patch test sensitization etc., current textbooks are recommended (Fisher, 1986; Adams and Fischer, 1990; Wahlberg, 1995).

Screening Series

To evaluate the significance of occupational exposures several screening series are available (Table 4.4). These extensive series, some containing more

Table 4.4 Some commercially available screening series of patch test allergens

Chemotechnique (1994/95)	Hermal (1994)
Bakery series	Antimicrobials, preservatives, antioxidants
Corticosteroid series	Cosmetics
Cosmetic series	Dental materials
Dental screening	Hairdressing
Epoxy series	Medicaments
Fragrance series	Metal compounds
Hairdressing series	Metalworking/technical oils
Isocyanate series	Perfumes, flavours
Medicament series	Pesticides
(Meth) acrylate series	Photographic chemicals
(Adhesives, dental and other)	Plants, woods
(Meth) acrylate series	Plastics, glues
(Nails – artificial)	Rubber chemicals
(Meth) acrylate series	Textile dyes
(Printing)	Vehicles, emulsifiers
Oil and cooling fluid series	
Photographic chemicals series	
Plant series	
Plastics and glues series	
Rubber additives series	
Shoe series	
Sunscreen series	
Textile colours and finish	

than 30 allergens, can be considered to cover the present exposure situation and are compiled from the experience gathered at departments of dermatology and occupational dermatology, and from the literature. Newly-defined allergens are added regularly.

Tests with the Patient's Working Materials and Products

To a department of occupational dermatology patients often bring suspected products and materials from their work environment. There are usually one or two ingredients of a product that are of interest as suspected allergens, while the rest are well-known non-allergenic chemicals. One can usually rely on documented information for the choice of vehicle and concentration if the suspected agents are available from suppliers of patch test allergens (Hermal, 1994; Chemotechnique, 1994/95). If one suspects that impurities or contaminants have caused the dermatitis, this can be discovered only by patch testing with samples of the ingredient obtained from the manufacturer or with samples from the actual batch. When testing, for example, paints or cutting fluids, unused products must be tested for comparison. Besides that, one risks overlooking true allergens by using overdiluted materials for testing. Solid products such as wood, paper, rubber, plants, textiles can usually be tested without modification or applied as extracts (water, acetone, ether, ethanol).

With an entirely new substance, where toxicological data are insufficient or absent, one has to consider the risk of complications. One can start with an open test and, if this is negative, continue with ordinary occlusive patch testing. Most allergens are tested in the concentration range of 0.01–10 per cent (Wahlberg, 1995). The usual recommendation is to start with a low concentration and then increase it when the preceding test is negative. If the test with a new substance is positive in a particular patient, one has to demonstrate in at least 10–20 unexposed controls that the actual test preparation is non-irritant (Fregert, 1985). Otherwise the observed reaction does not confirm allergenicity. At the author's clinic at least one new contact allergen is discovered each year when patch testing with materials provided by patients.

In Vitro *Testing for Diagnosing Contact Allergy*

In vitro test methods for diagnosing contact allergy have been reviewed by van Blomberg-van der Flier *et al.* (1989) and by McMillan and Burrows (1995). There are still problems of standardization, reproducibility, sensitivity, specificity, solubility of test substances. So far, mainly standard allergens have been studied *in vitro* (nickel, cobalt, chromium, formalin, urushiol), but one can anticipate even greater methodological problems with less defined occupational contact allergens (impurities, contaminants). In the standard, *in vivo*, patch test, 30–40 allergens, including the mixes, are studied simultaneously (Table 4.3), while with an *in vitro* test method only one allergen at a time is studied (see Chapter 9).

Most scientists agree that there is a long way to go before *in vitro* testing can replace standard patch testing in the clinic. The diagnosis of contact allergy will continue for some time to rely on the skill of the clinician, combined with *in vivo* analysis.

Chemical Investigations

Various chemical tests have been developed to detect the presence of contact allergens in both occupational and household products, and simple methods are available for nickel, chromate, formaldehyde, epoxy, atranorin and textile dyes (Wall, 1995).

A positive patch test reaction might be interpreted as 'unexplained' until the presence of the corresponding allergen can be demonstrated in the product(s) to which the patient was exposed prior to the appearance of dermatitis. For those individuals already sensitized, it is essential to avoid re-exposure to products containing allergen. In cases where the ingredient labelling is incomplete or unreliable, chemical investigations can be of great help. More advanced chemical methods have been used when detecting and defining the allergens in the epoxy system (Thorgeirsson, 1977), in phenol-formaldehyde resin (Bruze, 1985) and in colophony (Karlberg, 1988).

Use Tests, Repeated Open Application Test

The original use tests were intended to mimic the actual in use situation (repeated open applications to the skin) of a formulated product such as a cutting fluid, a paint, a shampoo, or a cosmetic cream. A positive outcome of the test supported the suspicion that the product in question had caused the patient's dermatitis. The primary goal was to reproduce the dermatitis – not to clarify its nature (allergic or irritant). These tests are now used increasingly to evaluate the clinical relevance of positive patch test reactions to ingredients of formulated products. The concentration of the particular ingredient seems to be so low that one may question whether the positive reaction at patch testing can explain the patient's dermatitis.

The repeated open application test (ROAT) in its present form was introduced by Hannuksela and Salo (1986). Commercial products in unmodified form, or patch test allergens, are applied twice daily for 7 days to the outer aspect of the upper arm, antecubital fossa or back skin (scapular area). An eczematous dermatitis – evaluated as a positive response – usually appears after 2–4 days of treatment.

The observed dermatitis may be due to contact allergy to an ingredient of a formulated product, but irritancy from other ingredients must be considered also. It is therefore recommended to use two coded samples simultaneously, one containing the allergen and one without (left versus right comparison). If there is a positive response only at the test site where the allergen-containing product has been applied, this strongly supports the assumption that the initial patch test reaction is relevant. On the other hand, reactions of the same intensity at both test sites are interpreted as an expression of irritancy.

Exposure Chamber

Exposure chambers may be used to study the effects on lung function, mucous membranes, and on the skin, of exposure to airborne allergens and irritants. The methodology for controlled provocation tests with airborne skin allergens and irritants is very limited. Reliable methods are lacking for the calculation of the skin-exposure dose to particles. An exposure chamber for the development of technique for controlled, occupational exposure of human skin to particles and gases has been built by our department (Lidén, personal communication).

Workplace Visits

The value of workplace visits in unexplained cases of work-related contact dermatitis is acknowledged (Rycroft, 1995). In our experience many cases are not explained or solved until we have seen the worker in the actual work situation. The exposure can be detailed, the degree of skin contamination evaluated and samples from working materials, gloves and cleansing agents etc. can be assembled for further testing and analysis.

Diagnoses and Differential Diagnoses

The diagnosis of a work-related allergic contact dermatitis is based mainly and traditionally on the demonstration of a positive patch test reaction. However, other essential factors known to support the diagnosis are: knowledge of exposure, localization of skin lesions, their morphology, demonstration of the presence of allergen in products and materials ('relevant exposure'), use tests, effect of treatment, avoidance of exposure and other preventive measures, and clinical course. Some of these aspects are discussed in more detail below. Especially for hand eczema, there are several alternative diagnoses (Table 4.2) and the clinician will also meet 'mixed' forms where the relative importance of a diagnosed contact allergy is hard to judge. It is the skill and experience of the dermatologist that is decisive for the outcome. In the author's experience, too much emphasis is put on an observed positive patch test reaction.

Specific Occupational Hazards

The presence of and exposure to allergens, irritants and chemicals causing contact urticaria in specified jobs are reviewed in some textbooks (Fregert, 1981; Adams, 1990; Rycroft, 1995). In the most extensive review (Adams, 1990) one can find – based on case reports and epidemiological studies – information on, in alphabetical order, agricultural workers, air hammer operators, anodizers etc. in more than 80 different occupations. In Table 4.5 an example is presented of what can be compiled from these textbooks concerning one profession – agricultural workers. These lists can be of great value when examining and questioning a patient. However, one has to be aware that the exposure in a trade is not constant; new chemicals and

Table 4.5 Exposure to contact allergens in agricultural workers

Fregert (1981)
Sensitizers: Rubber (boots, gloves, milking machines), cement, paints, local remedies for veterinary use, wood preservatives, plants, pesticides, antibiotics and preservatives in animal feed (quindoxin, ethoxyquine) penicillin for mastitis, cobalt in animal feed

Adams (1990)
Listed are:
19 standard allergens
30 additional allergens
More than 70 other chemicals and products, i.e. plants, pesticides, fumigants, feed additives, animal repellents

Rycroft (1995)
Sensitizers: Rubber (boots, gloves, milking machines), cement, plants, pesticides, wood preservatives, fertilizers (nickel, cobalt), soil disinfectants, animal feed additives (antibiotics, cobalt, vitamin K3, ethoxyquin, quinoxaline and derivates, dinitolmide, phenothiazines), veterinary medicaments

Compiled from some textbooks in order to demonstrate various degrees of completeness.

products are introduced, others disappear and some were initially introduced in a quite different job.

Treatment

Occupational allergic contact dermatitis is treated according to the same principles as non-occupational dermatitis. Besides topical treatment, peroral drugs such as corticosteroids and antihistamines, UV treatment, phototherapy, immunomodulators etc., much effort is applied to avoid relapses due to renewed occupational exposure. Preventive measures are described in more detail below and in Table 4.6.

Hardening or specific 'hyposensitization' is a controversial matter. It has been shown that workers exposed to contact allergens developed contact dermatitis, and were patch test positive, but could nevertheless continue their work without relapses. When re-tested they were no longer patch test positive – an indication of 'hardening'. However, to prove that specific hardening has taken place, stricter criteria should be applied (Wahlberg, 1992).

Prognosis

The overall medical prognosis for occupational contact dermatitis is poor (Fregert, 1975; Wall and Gebauer, 1991; Rosen and Freeman, 1993;

Table 4.6 Prevention of occupational allergic contact dermatitis

Chemicals
  Identification of allergens
  Occurrence, concentration of allergens in the work environment
  Allergen removal or replacement
  Modification or inactivation of allergens
  Predictive testing: sensitizing potential
Individual identified at pre-employment examination
  Those with increased susceptibility or predisposition
  Patients with a history of contact dermatitis
Avoidance of direct contact with products and materials
  Protective gloves
  Aprons, sleeves, boots, glasses, masks, etc.
  Protective (barrier) creams
  Automation, closed systems
  Efficient ventilation
Skin care programme
  Soaps, detergents, cleansing agents (allergen-free)
  Hot water, shower, sauna
  Soft towers
  Emollient and moisturizing creams
Miscellaneous
  Legislation
  Labelling of products and chemicals, safety sheets
  Information to patients, workers, supervisors
  Training of workers in special industrial processes
  Good housekeeping
  Research on prevention; dissemination of results obtained

Wrangsjö and Meding, 1994). It is recommended that outcome should be assessed as 'cured', 'improved' or 'not cured' to facilitate comparison between various measures such as changing duties or jobs, allergen avoidance, protective measures, for example, gloves (Table 4.6).

A significant difference exists in the prognoses of workers with different allergies. The improvement rate for allergy to p-phenylenediamine (a hairdressing allergen) is above 90 per cent, whilst the improvement rate for potassium dichromate is about 41 per cent ($p<0.001$) (Rosen and Freeman, 1993).

When comparing the prognoses of allergic contact dermatitis with those of irritant contact dermatitis one obtains controversial findings. If the allergens could be identified and eliminated from the patient's environment one would anticipate a better prognosis. Thus, the outcome of allergy to epoxy resins has been reported as favourable. The failure concerning chromate allergy is well-known and since we lack explanations this entity is said to be 'self-perpetuating'.

Prevention

The importance of disease prevention is evident and for human, social and economic reasons it would be of great benefit if workers exposed to allergenic chemicals and products could be protected from developing contact dermatitis.

The responsibility for *primary prevention*, i.e. prevention of the induction and onset of contact dermatitis, rests mainly with manufacturers and producers of products, with government agencies, consumer organizations, and in a factory with physicians, nurses and safety engineers. For *secondary prevention*, i.e. prevention of relapses, greater responsibility is placed on physicians treating the cases (industrial physicians, dermatologists), and on nurses and safety engineers in industry.

Essential preventive measures concerning occupational allergic contact dermatitis are listed in Table 4.6. All should be considered, and in the present author's experience the best results are achieved when several of the recommended prophylactic measures are combined. It is definitively less effective to rely on just one recommendation. To demonstrate that the suggested methods and measures are efficacious and cost-effective is a challenge to those involved in preventive dermatology. For example, current protective gloves are not perfect (Mellström *et al.*, 1994). Some are permeable to various chemicals, including contact allergens, and do not provide the promised protection. Side effects such as irritancy, latex allergy and contact allergy to rubber chemicals are common and discourage exposed workers from their use.

In our preventive strategy we recommend concentrating efforts on those allergens that cause the greatest frequency of occupational allergic contact dermatitis (Table 4.7) and cases of disablement.

Contact Allergy in the Normal Population

Case reports on contact allergy to new as well as to previously known allergens are presented from dermatological clinics and from departments of occupational dermatology, where a highly selected population has been examined. Such reports alert dermatologists, and if the observations are confirmed at other clinics and in other countries the size and the severity of the problem can be quantified.

However, more emphasis has recently been placed on the occurrence of contact allergy in the normal population, i.e. people with no history of skin complaints or skin disease. An example is given in Table 4.7, where 567 Danes from an unselected population were patch tested with a series of 23 haptens (Nielsen and Menné, 1992). It is clear, therefore, that positive patch test reactions are not uncommon in the normal population and this must be borne in mind when a positive reaction is found in a dermatitis patient. For

Table 4.7 Distribution of contact sensitization to 10 haptens and mixtures of haptens in an unselected Danish normal population (Nielsen and Menné, 1992) and in patients at the Department of Occupational Dermatology, Karolinska Hospital, Stockholm 1993–94

| | Distribution of contact sensitization (percentage positive) | | | |
| | Normal population | | Occupational patients | |
Hapten	Men ($n = 279$)	Women ($n = 288$)	Men ($n = 251$)	Women ($n = 328$)
Nickel sulfate	2.2	11.1	7.7	32.8
Fragrance mix	1.1	1.0	6.4	10.0
Balsam of Peru	0.7	1.4	3.2	7.3
Cobalt chloride	0.7	1.4	5.2	5.9
p-t-Butylphenolformaldehyde resin	1.1	1.0	2.8	1.5
Colophony	0.4	1.0	3.2	9.2
Isothiazolinones	0.4	1.0	2.4	1.5
Potassium dichromate	0.7	0.3	6.9	5.2
Epoxy resin	0.4	0.7	2.8	1.2
Thiuram mix	0.7	0.3	2.0	3.4

comparison, figures from the author's clinic are presented, from patch testing a selected group of patients with work-related dermatitis (Table 4.7).

Additional studies of the same kind as the Danish one are highly desirable to keep the reported frequency of positive patch test reactions in contact dermatitis patients in perspective. Such studies are, however, expensive, time-consuming and might cause ethical problems.

Classification of Contact Allergens

Definite Contact Allergens

We recently (Knudsen *et al.*, 1993) attempted to define 'definite contact allergens'. Our proposal was that, to be considered as a 'definite contact allergen':

1. The chemical has caused allergic contact dermatitis in at least one exposed person.

2. In this exposed person (or persons), a patch test with the analytically well defined chemical has produced a clearly positive reaction.

3. Patch tests with serial dilutions of the chemical compound have shown a dose-response relationship.

4. The chemical does not cause irritant reactions when tested in a statistically sufficient number of non-exposed persons. Bioavailable quantities relevant to the patch test concentrations should be used.
5. Patch testing should not be carried out in patients with current eczema and labile skin. If this has not been possible initially, the positive patch test must be repeated when the contact dermatitis has subsided considerably.

If these criteria were applied to the 3700 contact allergens reported by de Groot (1994) some would no doubt be rejected.

Significant Contact Allergens

Significant contact allergens are presumed to be able to cause allergic contact dermatitis in a substantial number of persons. The criteria used by the IARC (International Agency for Research on Cancer) to evaluate data on the carcinogenicity of chemicals is applied to contact allergens, i.e. human evidence, evidence from animal experiments (guinea pigs, mice), and other supporting evidence (quantitative structure-activity relationship (QSAR), *in vitro* experiments). The available information is validated, the combined evidence considered and the chemical classified into one of the following groups:

Group 1:   The chemical causes allergic contact dermatitis to a significant degree in man. This category is used only when there is sufficient human evidence.

Group 2A: The chemical probably causes allergic contact dermatitis to a significant degree in man. This category is used when there is limited human evidence and sufficient evidence in animals. Occasionally, strong supporting evidence may replace human evidence, for example structural similarity to other allergens for which there is human evidence.

Group 2B: The chemical may possibly cause allergic contact dermatitis to a significant degree in man. This category is used when there is sufficient evidence in animals and no human data. It can be used also in some cases when limited evidence from animals and limited or inadequate human data are available, especially when there is additional supporting evidence.

Group 3:   The available data does not allow classification of the chemical as to its degree of sensitizing potential.

Group 4:   The chemical is not a significant contact sensitizer and does not cause allergic contact dermatitis in a substantial number of persons. Classification in this category requires sufficient human evidence and many years of experience with the substance.

Chemicals classified in group 1, 2A and 2B are classified as significant human contact allergens. Application of these proposed criteria would probably reduce the number of contact allergens the dermatologist has to administer, 3700 allergens being far too many to handle effectively. A constructive discussion of criteria would be greatly welcomed.

The Future

We conclude with a brief list of future hopes and needs.

1. Reliable methods of quantifying skin contamination by contact allergens in industry.
2. Additional, simple spot-tests to demonstrate the presence of allergens in products.
3. Ingredient labelling – ingredients in concentrations <1.0 per cent should also be stated.
4. A simple, quick and reproducible *in vitro* test method for diagnosing contact allergy.
5. Consensus on the classification of contact allergens.
6. Particulars of the occurrence of contact allergy in the normal population.

References

ADAMS, R.M. (ed.), 1990, *Occupational Skin Disease*, 2nd Edn, Philadelphia, London, Toronto, Montreal, Sydney, Tokyo: W.B. Saunders Company.

ADAMS, R.M. and FISCHER, T., 1990, Diagnostic patch testing, in Adams, R.M. (ed.) *Occupational Skin Disease*, 2nd Edn, pp. 223–53, Philadelphia, London, Toronto, Montreal, Sydney, Tokyo: W.B. Saunders Company.

BRUZE, M., 1985, Contact sensitizers in resins based on phenol and formaldehyde, *Thesis, Acta. Derm. Venereol. Suppl. (Stockh.)*, **119**, 1–83.

CHEMOTECHNIQUE, 1994/95, *Patch Test Allergens*.

DE GROOT, A.C., 1986, *Patch Testing*, Amsterdam, New York, Oxford: Elsevier.

1994, *Patch Testing*, 2nd Edn, Amsterdam, London, New York, Tokyo: Elsevier.

FISHER, A.A., 1986, The role of patch testing, in Fisher, A.A. (ed.), *Contact Dermatitis*, 3rd Edn, pp. 9–29, Philadelphia: Lea & Febiger.

FREGERT, S., 1975, Occupational dermatitis in a 10-year material, *Contact Dermatitis*, **1**, 96–107.

1981, *Manual of Contact Dermatitis*, 2nd Edn, Copenhagen: Year Book, Medical Publishers, Inc.

1985, Publication of allergens, *Contact Dermatitis*, **12**, 123–4.

FROSCH, P.J. and RYCROFT, R.J.G., 1995, International legal aspects of contact dermatitis, in Rycroft, R.J.G., Mennë, T. and Frosch, P.J. (eds.) *Textbook of Contact Dermatitis*, pp. 751–68, Berlin, Heidelberg, New York: Springer-Verlag.

GRIFFITH, J.F. and BUEHLER, E.V., 1977, Prediction of skin irritancy and sensitizing potential by testing with animals and man, in Drill, V.A. and Lazar, P. (eds.) *Cutaneous Toxicity*, pp. 155–73, New York, San Francisco, London: Academic Press Inc.

GRIFFITHS, W.A.D., 1985, Industrial dermatitis – a national problem, in Griffiths, W.A.D. and Wilkinson, D.S. (eds.) *Essentials of Industrial Dermatology*, pp. 1–11. Oxford, London, Edinburgh, Boston, Palo Alto, Melbourne: Blackwell Scientific Publications.

HANNUKSELA, M. and SALO, H., 1986, The repeated open application test (ROAT), *Contact Dermatitis*, **14**, 221–7.

HERMAL. TROLAB, 1994, *Patch test allergens.*

JADASSOHN, J., 1896, Zur Kenntnis der medikamentösen Dermatosen, Verhandlungen der Deutschen Dermatologischen Gesellschaft, pp. 106, *Fünfter Kongress, Raz*, 1895. Braunmuller, Vienna.

KARLBERG, A-T., 1988, Contact allergy to colophony. Chemical identification of allergens, sensitization experiments and clinical experiences, *Thesis, Karolinska Institute*, Stockholm, Sweden, 1–43.

KLIGMAN, A.M., 1966, The identification of contact allergens by human assay. III. The maximization test. A procedure for screening and rating contact sensitizers, *J. Invest. Dermatol.*, **47**, 393–409.

KNUDSEN, B.B., WAHLBERG, J.E., ANDERSEN, I. and MENNÈ, T., 1993, Classification of contact allergens, *Dermatosen in Beruf und Umwelt.*, **41**, 5–9.

MARZULLI, F.N. and MAIBACH, H.I., 1973, Antimicrobials: Experimental contact sensitization in man, *J. Soc. Cosmet. Chem.*, **24**, 399–421.

MATHIAS, C.G.T., 1985, The cost of occupational skin disease, *Arch. Dermatol.*, **121**, 332–4.

MCMILLAN, C. and BURROWS, D. 1995, In vitro testing in contact hypersensitivity, in Rycroft, R.J.G., Menné, T. and Frosch, P.J. (eds.) *Textbook of Contact Dermatitis*, 2nd Edn, pp. 306–22, Berlin, Heidelberg, New York: Springer-Verlag.

MELLSTRÖM, G.A., WAHLBERG, J.E. and MAIBACH, H.I., 1994, *Protective Gloves for Occupational Use*, Boca Raton: CRC Press, Inc.

NIELSEN, N.H. and MENNÉ, T., 1992, Allergic contact sensitization in an unselected Danish population, *Acta Derm. Venereol. (Stockh.)*, **72**, 456–60.

ROSEN, R.H. and FREEMAN, S., 1993, Prognosis of occupational contact dermatitis in New South Wales, Australia, *Contact Dermatitis*, **29**, 88–93.

RYCROFT, R.J.G., 1995, Occupational contact dermatitis, in Rycroft, R.J.G., Mennè, T. and Frosch, P.J. (eds.) *Textbook of Contact Dermatitis*, 2nd Edn, pp. 343–400, Berlin, Heidelberg, New York: Springer-Verlag.

THORGEIRSSON, A., 1977, Sensitization capacity of epoxy resin compounds. Thesis, *University of Lund*, Sweden, 1–28.

VON BLOMBERG-VAN DER FLIER, B.M.E., BRUYNZEEL, D.P. and SCHEPER, R.J., 1989, Impact of 25 years of in vitro testing in allergic contact dermatitis, in Frosch, P.J., Dooms-Goossens, A., Lachapelle, J.-M., Rycroft, R.J.G. and Scheper, R.J. (eds.) *Current Topics in Contact Dermatitis*, pp. 569–77, Berlin, Heidelberg, New York: Springer-Verlag.

WAHLBERG, J.E., 1992, Hardening. Letter to the Editor, *Contact Dermatitis*, **26**, 359.

WAHLBERG, J.E., 1995, Patch testing, in Rycroft, R.J.G., Menné, T. and Frosch, P.J. (eds.) *Textbook of Contact Dermatitis*, 2nd Edn, p.p. 241–68, Berlin,

Berlin, Heidelberg, New York: Springer-Verlag.

WALL, L.M., 1995, Spot tests and chemical analyses for allergen evaluation, in Rycroft, R.J.G., Menné, T. and Frosch, P.J. (eds.) *Textbook of Contact Dermatitis*, 2nd Edn, pp. 277–85, Berlin, Heidelberg, New York: Springer-Verlag.

WALL, L.M. and GEBAUER, K.A., 1991, A follow-up study of occupational skin disease in Western Australia, *Contact Dermatitis*, **24**, 241–3.

WRANGSJÖ, K. and MEDING, B., 1994, Occupational contact allergy to rubber chemicals, *Dermatosen*, **42**, 184–9.

5

Chemical Aspects of Contact Hypersensitivity

M.D. BARRATT and D.A. BASKETTER

Unilever Environmental Safety Laboratory, Sharnbrook

Introduction

The correlation of the protein reactivity of chemicals with their skin sensitization potential is well established (Dupuis and Benezra, 1982; Basketter and Roberts, 1990) It is self evident, therefore, that if a chemical is capable of reacting with a protein either directly or after appropriate (bio)chemical transformation, then it has the potential to be a contact allergen. The potential of a chemical to act as a contact allergen is further modulated by its ability to penetrate the skin; this is apparent from a number of quantitative structure-activity relationship (QSAR) studies (Basketter *et al.*, 1992; Barratt *et al.*, 1994b) in which skin sensitization potential has been found to depend crucially on parameters such as $\log P$, which have also been found to be equally important determinants of percutaneous absorption (Flynn, 1990).

We review here the ways in which consideration of the chemistry of contact allergy can contribute to its better understanding and also provide an opportunity to identify potential contact allergens without recourse to animal testing.

Chemistry/Mechanisms

There is a well-established correlation between the ability of chemicals to react with proteins to form covalently linked conjugates and their skin sensitization potential (Dupuis and Benezra, 1982). It is worth mentioning at this stage that the great majority of protein-reactive chemicals are electrophilic in nature. This section reviews some of the more important reactions of organic chemicals with proteins, which have been identified as leading to contact allergy. For simplicity, these reactions have been grouped together by mechanism; the same mechanistic groups are used in the later section devoted to expert systems. Examples of chemicals or groups of chemicals which are postulated to sensitize via the various chemical reaction types are shown in Scheme 5.1.

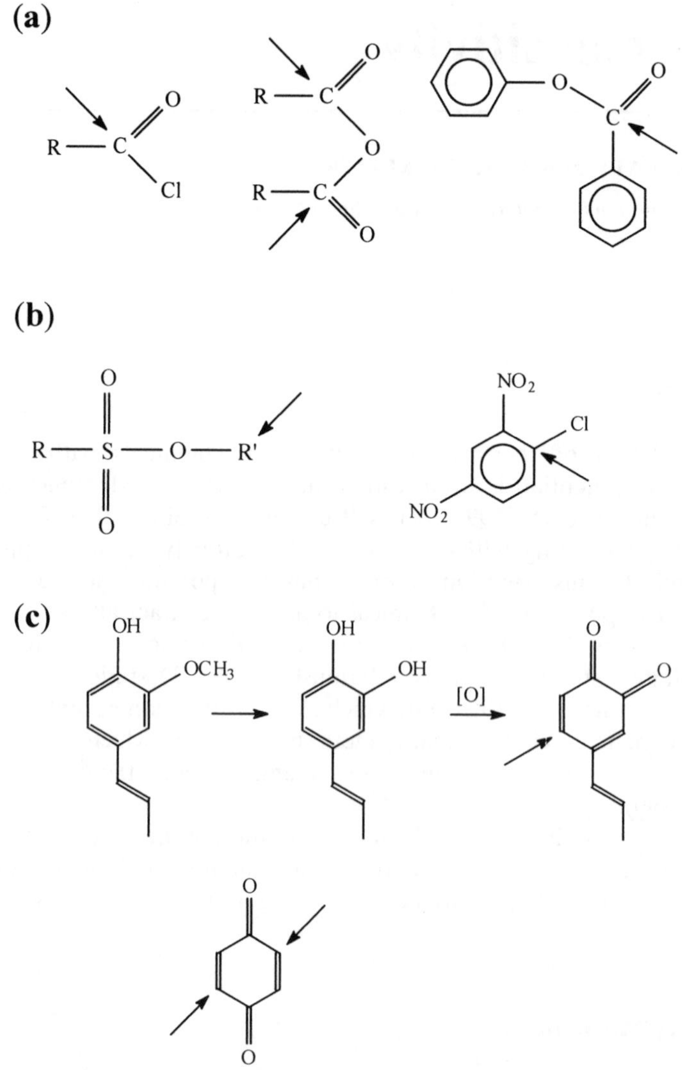

(a)

(b)

(c)

Scheme 5.1 Examples of chemicals or groups of chemicals by reaction type; (a) acylating agents, (b) alkylating/arylating agents, (c) Michael electrophiles and precursors, (d) aldehydes and precursors, (e) free radical generators, (f) thiol exchange agents. Postulated sites for reaction with protein nucleophiles are indicated by arrows

(d)

$$R—CH{=}O \qquad \underset{H}{\overset{R}{\diagdown}}C\underset{OCH_3}{\overset{OCH_3}{\diagup}} \longrightarrow R—CH{=}O$$

(e)

CH$_3$ ... SO$_2$ ... NHNa $\xrightarrow{H^+}$ CH$_3$ ... SO$_2$ ... NH$_2$ $\longrightarrow$ CH$_3$ ... SO$_2$ ... NH$^\bullet$

OCH$_3$ $\longrightarrow$ OH $\xrightarrow{[O]}$ O $\longrightarrow$ O

(f)

R—SH $\qquad$ R—S-S—R $\qquad$ CH$_2${=}CH—CH$_2$—S—S—CH$_2$—CH{=}CH$_2$

Acylating Agents

Acylating agents comprise a large and important group of contact allergens which includes acid anhydrides and halides, phenyl esters and some ring-strained esters, amides, thioesters and thioamides. All of these chemicals possess the ability to react with the ϵ-amino group of lysine residues in proteins to form amide derivatives.

Acid halides and anhydrides have long been known to be strong skin sensitizers in the guinea pig (Landsteiner and Jacobs, 1936; Chase, 1947). Phenyl esters were recognized as skin sensitizers more recently (Marchand *et al.*, 1982) and have also been the subject of a QSAR study (Barratt *et al.*, 1994b). The best-known examples of sensitizing ring-strained amides and esters are the penicillins such as penicillin G (Kligman, 1966; Guillot *et al.*, 1983) and β-propiolactone (Ashby *et al.*, 1993).

Alkylating/Arylating Agents

As with acylating agents, this group encapsulates a large number of chemicals with different functional groups, some of the commonest being alkyl halides, sulphates and sulphonates and reactive aromatic halo-compounds. Reactions with both ε-amino group of lysine residues and thiol groups of cysteine in proteins are presumably possible. Amongst the alkyl halides, skin sensitization from substituted benzyl chlorides has been reported (Rao *et al.*, 1981) and the sensitization potential of a homologous series of alkyl bromides in the local lymph node assay (LLNA; see Chapter 8) have been the subject of a QSAR study (Basketter *et al.*, 1992). A QSAR study has been carried out on the sensitization of alkyl alkane sulphonates in the guinea pig (Roberts and Basketter, 1990). Alkane and alkene sultones (Roberts and Williams, 1983), the latter being some of the most potent contact allergens yet encountered, are also members of the alkyl sulphonate family. 2,4-Dinitrochlorobenzene, probably one of the best known and most widely used experimental contact allergens (Goodwin *et al.*, 1981; Friedman and Moss, 1985), is an example of a reactive aromatic halo-compound.

Michael Electrophiles and Precursors

The Michael reaction involving the addition of nucleophiles across α,β-unsaturated carbonyl compounds plays a role in the reactivity of a large number of skin sensitizers; these chemicals include α,β-unsaturated esters, aldehydes, ketones and amides. Michael electrophiles frequently occur as the oxidation products of chemicals of plant origin, and are responsible for a number of contact allergies, perhaps the best known and most investigated of these being poison ivy (Liberato *et al.*, 1981). The role of the Michael reaction in contact dermatitis to plants was studied extensively by the late Claude Benezra (Benezra *et al.*, 1985; Benezra and Epstein, 1986; Benezra and Ducombs, 1987). Examples of common chemicals which sensitize directly via this mechanism are acrylate esters, acrylamides and acrolein.

One chemical which is sometimes mistakenly cited as reacting either with protein or DNA via a Michael reaction is the α,β-unsaturated cyclic ester, coumarin. Although α,β-unsaturated esters with an aromatic substituent in the β-position, for example cinnamate esters, undergo Michael reactions with carbanions in anhydrous ethanol, the overwhelming body of evidence suggests that they do not add to the nucleophilic groups on proteins. This presumably results from the weak electron-donating properties of the aromatic ring. Cinnamate esters and coumarin are well known as being non-sensitizing, indeed many tonnes of the former are spread over people's bodies annually in the form of sunscreens. In contrast to coumarin, dihydrocoumarin is a skin sensitizer and may well react via the phenyl ester acylation route. Coumarin is also a phenyl ester, but can be expected to be less reactive since cinnamic acid is a weaker acid than β-phenylpropionic acid and therefore will be a poorer leaving group; the lactone ring system in coumarin is also likely to be stabilized through conjugation of the double bond with the aromatic ring.

As mentioned above, some sensitizers in this category are generated by the oxidation of other chemicals which are not themselves sensitizing. The oxidation of catechols and hydroquinones respectively to *ortho-* and *para-*quinones are well-known examples of such chemicals. This oxidation process can occur either before or after contact and penetration through the skin. This mechanism has been modelled in a detailed electron spin resonance study (Davies *et al.*, 1995) using 4-methylcatechol, a known skin sensitizer (Barratt and Basketter, 1992); oxidation to the orthoquinone was followed by addition of model nucleophiles (hydroxide and methoxide ions) to the 3- and 5-position respectively. For some chemicals, skin metabolism may occur to remove a 'protecting' group from a phenolic hydroxyl before oxidation can take place. In the case of isoeugenol, there is evidence that the O-methyl group is removed in the skin prior to oxidation to give a sensitizing *ortho*-quinone (Barratt and Basketter, 1992).

Aldehydes and Precursors

A number of simple aldehydes are known to be skin sensitizers, e.g. formaldehyde, butyraldehyde and benzaldehyde (see de Groot *et al*, 1994); aromatic aldehydes are less reactive than aliphatic aldehydes, due to the electron-donating (deactivating) properties of the aromatic ring. Reaction of aldehydes with proteins is assumed generally to proceed via Schiff's base formation between the aldehyde carbonyl group and an ϵ-amino group of a lysine residue. Stabilization of this linkage by biochemical reduction is then a possibility.

Some precursors of aldehydes are also known to be skin sensitizers. These include acetals such as phenylacetaldehyde dimethyl acetal and ethylidene heptanoate acetate and formaldehyde donors, e.g. dimethylol-5, 5-dimethyl-hydantoin and imidazolidinyl urea (Cronin and Basketter, 1994). Release of the reactive aldehydes from these chemicals can occur either through metabolism or simply by slow hydrolysis at physiological pH.

Free Radical Generators

Whereas allergic responses from the reaction of free radicals are widespread in photoallergy, for example fentichlor, bithionol and musk ambrette (Pendlington and Barratt, 1990; Motten *et al.*, 1983), only a few examples have been identified in contact allergy. Free radicals generated from the allergen chloramine-T under mildly acidic conditions (Evans *et al.*, 1985) have been implicated in its covalent reaction with proteins (Evans *et al.*, 1986) and recent studies have shown that radical reactions are involved in hapten binding to proteins by some hydroperoxides (Gäfvert *et al.*, 1994; Lepoittevin and Karlberg, 1994).

A 'phenolic radical mechanism' has been postulated for the reaction of a number of phenols with proteins (Barratt and Basketter, 1992). This mechanism is initiated by the abstraction of a hydrogen atom from the hydroxyl group of the phenol. The free radicals formed react via their mesomeric forms, primarily at the position *ortho* to the hydroxyl. Eugenol, 4-hydroxystilbene, 4-allylanisole and anethole are all believed to react via this mechanism, the latter two after the metabolic removal of protecting O-methyl groups. A somewhat wider involvement of free radical mechanisms in the generation of haptens is proposed by Schmidt *et al.* (1990).

Thiol-Exchange Agents

A number of chemicals containing disulphide groups are believed to react covalently with proteins via nucleophilic attack by protein thiol groups. Examples of sensitizers reacting via this mechanism are allyl propyl disulphide and diallyl disulphide (Papageorgiou *et al.*, 1983; Kaniwa *et al.*, 1992). A similar mechanism may also exist in which chemicals containing thiol groups can react with the cystine disulphide bridges of proteins.

Prohaptens and Skin Metabolism

As mentioned earlier, there is an important correlation between the protein reactivity of chemicals and their skin sensitization potential. A number of chemicals which are skin sensitizers do not react directly with skin proteins, but undergo activation or metabolism in the skin to acquire that reactivity; such chemicals are called prohaptens. In general, it is quite possible to make a reasonable prediction of the detailed mechanism via which a chemical causes skin sensitization, although this is usually much harder to prove in practice (Barratt and Basketter, 1992; Franot *et al.*, 1994). Before making predictions of any likely contact allergenic potential on the basis of the structure of a particular chemical, it is therefore necessary to consider also the extent to which that chemical may be changed before contact with, or by metabolism in or on, the skin.

There are many documented examples of prohaptens in skin sensitization. For instance, the important haptens in turpentine and colophony are formed by air oxidation (Hellerstrom *et al.*, 1955; Gäfvert *et al.*, 1994) as are those in *d*-limonene (Karlberg *et al.*, 1992). In these examples the new and reactive chemical species are almost certainly formed long before skin contact takes place. On the other hand there are chemicals which almost certainly require metabolic processes in the epidermis to produce the reactive species. Examples of the latter include chemically unreactive fragrance molecules such as isoeugenol and its derivatives where enzymatic demethylation appears to be the first step in the activation process (Barratt and Basketter, 1992). The resulting catechols are then oxidized to give reactive orthoquinones. The catechol, urushiol, which is the sensitizing component of poison ivy (Dupuis, 1979) is understood to undergo an identical oxidation step. Analogous pathways have also been proposed for the sensitization of paraquinones and their precursors (Mayer, 1954). The metabolic chemistry that produces the mutagenic and carcinogenic effects of some polyaromatic hydrocarbons, which are also skin sensitizers (Ashby *et al.*, 1993), is well documented. A similar mechanism is assumed for their skin sensitization potential, but has not yet been confirmed. However, there are many other molecules which are at first sight chemically unreactive, but which nevertheless do sensitize and thus for which some type of transformation to a reactive species must take place (Basketter and Lidén, 1992).

While it is not appropriate in this chapter to provide a detailed review of the metabolic capabilities of the skin, a number of reviews on the subject have been published in recent years (Martin *et al.*, 1987; Kao and Carver, 1990; Hotchkiss, 1992; Hotchkiss, 1995). These reviews suggest that skin has a wide ranging metabolic capacity which can perform essentially all of the metabolic transformations which are known to be carried out by the liver. Furthermore, as is the case with the liver, metabolizing enzymes in keratinocytes can be induced (Vecchini *et al.*, 1995), so that repeated skin contact with a chemical might be expected to result in altered handling compared with that encountered from a single exposure.

At present, knowledge of the actual role of metabolic processes in skin in the context of contact allergy is limited to a few instances, such as the enzymatic hydrolysis of glucosides from tulip bulbs to generate the sensitizing species (Bergman *et al.*, 1967). In postulating metabolic pathways for the skin, much use is made of what is known to take place in the liver; however attempts are now being made to explore this area. Evidence generated in our own laboratory suggests that sensitization to cinnamic alcohol is due to conversion to the aldehyde via the action of alcohol dehydrogenase (Basketter, 1992) and the role of P4501A in the metabolic conversion of eugenol and isoeugenol into reactive haptens in skin is under investigation (Scholes *et al.*, 1994). Nevertheless this area of research represents largely virgin territory.

Quantitative Structure Activity Relationships (QSARs)

The basis underlying the development of QSARs is that the properties of a chemical are inherent in its molecular structure. If the mechanistic link between the property of concern and the structure can be derived or postulated, this can be used to derive relevant parameters and a QSAR can, in principle, be established.

QSARs for skin sensitization are based on the concept that the key factors governing the magnitude of the sensitization response are the reactivity of the chemical, its ability to locate in the crucial epidermal environment (skin permeability) and the dose applied. It was this concept that led to the development of the Relative Alkylation Index (RAI) model (Roberts and Williams, 1982) which was used initially to provide equations describing the skin sensitizing properties of sultones. In general, RAI models use a modular dose and log of the octanol water partition coefficient as a skin permeability parameter. For a study of the sensitization potential of a series of long chain haloalkanes where skin penetration was limited by high hydrophobicity, a $-(\log P)^2$ term was found to be valuable (Basketter *et al.*, 1992). A similar relationship involving $-(\log P)^2$ has been found for the *in vitro* skin penetration of a series of phenols (Hinz *et al.*, 1991).

The chemical reactivity term can be rather difficult to obtain. In the cases of studies of the sensitization potential of diacrylates and methacrylates (Roberts, 1987) and alkyl transfer agents (Roberts and Basketter, 1990) it has been possible to make estimates. For the long chain haloalkanes work, it was not found to be an important variable (Basketter *et al.*, 1992); these examples, however, represent very restricted datasets. Possibly the best option, which was proposed in the original paper (Roberts and Williams, 1982), is to measure the chemical reactivity *in vitro* using a defined nucleophile (usually *n*-butylamine); this has been done recently for a family of furanone derivatives (Franot *et al.*, 1994a, b). Measurement of chemical reactivity, however, is time-consuming and difficult. The choice of acceptor nucleophile may be crucial which can be a problem since it is exceptional that we have any clue as to the nature of the important *in vivo* acceptor sites (Franot *et al.*, 1993).

In a recent QSAR investigation of the sensitization potential of a set of 3- and 4- substituted phenyl benzoates, a relationship was found which required neither dose nor reactivity (Barratt *et al.*, 1994). The total erythema score (TES) from testing these chemicals in the Modified Single Injection Adjuvant Test (Goodwin and Johnson, 1985), challenged at their maximum non-irritant concentrations, was found to have a positive dependence on log P and a negative dependence on molecular volume, these two parameters accounting for 85.5 per cent of the variance in the dataset. This is illustrated in Figure 5.1. In QSAR studies of skin permeability, log (human skin permeability coefficient) has been shown to increase with increasing log P and with decreasing molecular weight (Potts and Guy, 1992) or molecular volume (Barratt, 1995). In the phenyl benzoate study, no statistical dependence could

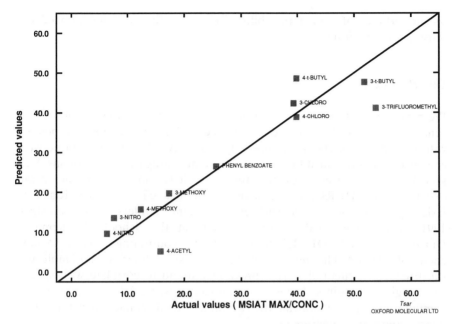

Figure 5.1 QSAR plot of actual versus predicted values of sensitization scores (TES) for 11 phenyl benzoates with different substituents on the phenol leaving group. TES = 26.48 clog $P - 0.394$ MV -6.673, $r^2 = 0.855$. Data ex Barratt *et al.*, 1994b

be found between the sensitization potential and the relative chemical reactivities of the chemicals; indeed, the two most reactive chemicals (nitrophenyl derivatives) proved to be the least sensitizing, presumably because they had low log P values and high molecular volumes.

From these few studies, it is clear that skin sensitization potential can be modelled, using parameters representing chemical reactivity, skin permeability and the dose applied. In practice, it may be possible to create models without the reactivity and/or dose parameters (these being implied in the nature of the dataset). The common feature of all these models is the presence of at least one parameter modelling skin permeability (usually log P).

Because almost all of the QSARs for skin sensitization developed to date are restricted to groups of chemicals with a well defined mode of action, often also belonging to homologous series, their value as tools for the prediction of skin sensitization potential is correspondingly limited. There is probably no 'general' QSAR for skin sensitization. This is reflected in two publications of QSAR models for the skin sensitization of heterogeneous groups of chemicals (Cronin and Basketter, 1994; Magee *et al.*, 1994), both of which employ the use of indicator variables to bring together chemicals reacting by different mechanistic pathways. The real value of QSAR models may be as an indicator of when our mechanistic understanding is sound, for example in confirming the importance of skin permeability factors for the determination of skin sensitization potential.

Expert Systems

We have demonstrated in previous sections that, despite the complexities of some of the metabolic processes which lead to skin sensitization, it is possible with the benefit of chemical knowledge to derive the relationship between chemical structure and ability to form covalent conjugates with proteins. Such knowledge relating chemical structure to toxicity can be programmed into expert systems. DEREK (an acronym for 'Deductive Estimation of Risk from Existing Knowledge') is one such expert system (Sanderson and Earnshaw, 1991), being developed by LHASA UK at the School of Chemistry, University of Leeds. DEREK embodies both a controlling programme and a chemical rulebase. The chemical rulebase consists of descriptions of molecular substructures 'structural alerts', previously found to correlate with specific toxicological endpoints. The user communicates with DEREK via interactive computer graphics by drawing the two-dimensional chemical structure of the query molecule on the screen.

Identification of Structural Alerts

Structural alerts for skin sensitization were derived initially from those chemicals within the Unilever historical database, which classified as strong or moderate sensitizers; these were the chemicals which currently would classify as skin sensitizers according to EC criteria (EEC, 1983). For this purpose, the chemicals were divided into groups either on the basis of reaction mechanisms or by empirical derivation:

acylating agents
alkylating/arylating agents
'Michael' electrophiles and precursors
aldehydes and precursors
free radical generators
'thiol-exchange' agents
others (empirical).

Forty rules (structural alerts) were identified from these groups of compounds and programmed into the DEREK system; these 40 structural alerts for skin sensitization have been published elsewhere (Barratt *et al.*, 1994a). The DEREK skin sensitization rulebase has now been extended to contain around 50 rules. Some of the more recent rules are shown in Figure 5.2.

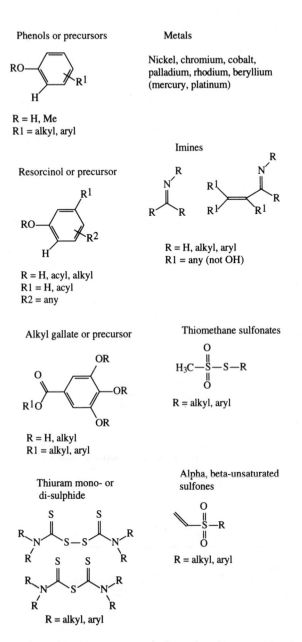

Phenols or precursors

R = H, Me
R1 = alkyl, aryl

Metals

Nickel, chromium, cobalt,
palladium, rhodium, beryllium
(mercury, platinum)

Imines

R = H, alkyl, aryl
R1 = any (not OH)

Resorcinol or precursor

R = H, acyl, alkyl
R1 = H, acyl
R2 = any

Alkyl gallate or precursor

R = H, alkyl
R1 = alkyl, aryl

Thiomethane sulfonates

R = alkyl, aryl

Thiuram mono- or
di-sulphide

R = alkyl, aryl

Alpha, beta-unsaturated
sulfones

R = alkyl, aryl

Figure 5.2 Examples of DEREK structural alerts for skin sensitization

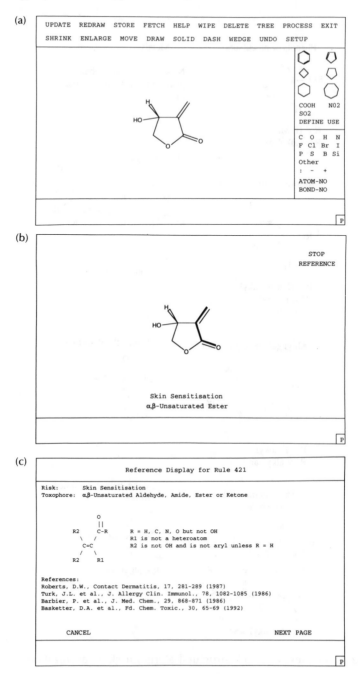

Figure 5.3 Typical screens from the DEREK system showing (a) a chemical structure prior to processing for structural alerts, (b) the structure with the structural alert identified and (c) the reference screen containing information about the rule which has been fired

Processing Structures Through DEREK

Typical screens from the DEREK system are shown in Figure 5.3. Of the 294 molecules in the database, 135 had sensitization scores such that they would be classified as sensitizers according to Annex V of the EC Dangerous Substances Directive (i.e. strong and moderate – at least 30 per cent of test guinea pigs positive) and 159 would not be classified as sensitizers (made up of 120 negative and 39 weak).

Of the 135 sensitizers, DEREK identifies structural alerts likely to lead to skin sensitization in 133. The two sensitizers not identified by the rulebase as containing structural alerts for skin sensitization are abietic acid and cinnamic alcohol. The sensitization potential of both chemicals is believed to arise from oxidation products, 7-oxodehydroabietic acid and 15-hydroxy-7-oxodehydroabietic acid in abietic acid (Karlberg, 1991), and cinnamic aldehyde in cinnamic alcohol (Basketter, 1992). Both of these sensitizing impurities trigger structural alerts in the DEREK system.

Of the 120 negative chemicals and the 39 weak sensitizers (chemicals showing some response but not classifying as sensitizers), the DEREK sensitization rulebase identified structural alerts respectively in 22 and 16 of the chemicals. The reason for these apparent 'false positives' lies in the fact that skin sensitization potential depends not just on the ability to react with a protein either directly or after appropriate (bio)chemical transformation, but also on its ability to penetrate the skin.

The Role of Skin Permeability

A chemical that does not penetrate skin cannot induce or elicit allergic contact dermatitis unless the dermal barrier is bypassed. The permeability of chemicals through the skin has been shown to depend on a few key physico-chemical characteristics. It is widely accepted that the skin permeability of a chemical increases with increasing lipophilicity, up to a point; it is also recognized that for chemicals with the same lipophilicity, smaller chemicals penetrate more readily than larger chemicals. Thus, it is clear that some chemicals may contain a structural alert for skin sensitization, but may fail to manifest that property because their skin permeability is too low.

As described above, the octanol-water partition coefficient (P) has been shown to be the most important parameter for modelling the skin permeability of chemicals (Flynn, 1990), higher log P values, i.e. greater lipophilicity broadly leading to greater permeability. Molecular size has been incorporated into models for skin permeability using the parameter molecular weight (Potts and Guy, 1992). A more recent treatment (Barratt, 1995) of the dataset published by Flynn (1990) uses molecular volume as the size parameter together with melting point as a measure of aqueous solubility (Suzuki, 1991).

Table 5.1 The effect of polarity on skin sensitization response

Chemical	Structural alert	Polarity	Sensitization response
4-Chloroaniline	Aromatic amine	Apolar	Strong
4-Aminobenzoate	Aromatic amine	Ionic	Weak/negative
Phenyl benzoate	Phenyl ester	Apolar	Strong
Sodium 4-benzoyloxybenzoate	Phenyl ester	Ionic	Weak/negative
Ethylene glycol dimethacrylate	α,β-Unsaturated ester	Apolar	Strong
2-Hydroxyethyl acrylate	α,β-Unsaturated ester	Polar	Negative

Examples of chemicals where differences in lipophilicity (or polarity) give rise to different sensitization responses are shown in Table 5.1. 4-Aminobenzoic acid (a zwitterionic compound), sodium 4-benzoyloxybenzoate and 2-hydroxyethyl methacrylate (moderately polar) are weak or non-sensitizers, whilst 4-chloroaniline, phenyl benzoate and ethylene glycol dimethacrylate are moderate or strong sensitizers. The former three chemicals are quite polar by virtue of possessing charged or polar groups and will thus penetrate the skin much less readily than the latter three chemicals.

Although still under development, the DEREK skin sensitization rulebase together with an assessment of the likely skin permeability of the chemical, forms part of the first step in a strategic approach to the identification of contact allergens.

The Role of Chemical Knowledge in Predictive Testing

A scheme illustrating a strategic approach to skin sensitization hazard identification, based on an understanding of the chemistry of allergic contact dermatitis, is shown in Scheme 5.2. A substance of defined chemical structure which is to be investigated is initially entered into the DEREK system. If no structural alert is identified, then although the chemical is unlikely to be a significant skin sensitizer, at present this should be confirmed using a standard animal assay; the LLNA (Kimber and Basketter, 1992; Kimber *et al.*, 1994) is considered most appropriate. When a skin sensitization structural alert is identified, the chemical has met one of the two criteria for classification as a skin sensitizer. However, to behave as a skin sensitiser, a chemical must be able to partition into the relevant skin compartment in addition to being able to derivatize skin protein.

In the next phase of this approach, a chemical which has been identified by DEREK as possessing a skin sensitization structural alert is evaluated in terms of its skin permeability using a QSAR model as described above. If the skin penetration of the chemical is judged to be sufficiently high, then it may be

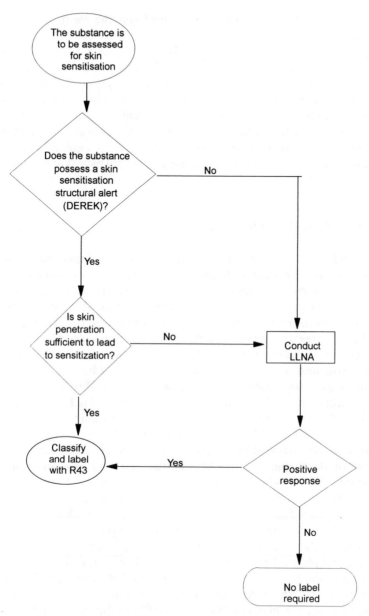

Scheme 5.2 A strategic approach to skin sensitization hazard identification

assumed also to have significant skin sensitization potential and can be classified and labelled accordingly. If skin penetration is judged to be insignificant, the chemical is considered unlikely to be a skin sensitizer. In the latter case and where the extent of skin penetration is judged to be moderate or equivocal, it is considered prudent to assess the chemical in a suitable animal model. Again, the LLNA is considered the most appropriate test method.

Whatever route is taken to trigger the conduct of a LLNA, the practical outcome is the same. If the chemical is positive in this assay, it should be classified as a skin sensitizer and labelled accordingly (EU, 1993). When the result clearly does not meet the criteria for classification, then in our view no further work should be necessary. The chemical may be regarded as having insufficient sensitization potential to merit classification and labelling as a skin sensitizer. Current regulations require evidence from a guinea pig maximization test as justification for not labelling a chemical as a skin sensitizer (EU, 1993).

Animal Welfare Considerations

The DEREK skin sensitization rulebase was developed originally from analysis of over 300 chemicals tested in the GPMT, approximately half of which would be classified and labelled as skin sensitizers according to current EU criteria (Barratt *et al.*, 1994a). With the exception of one or two chemicals which are sensitizers due to the presence of impurities, the DEREK rulebase identifies structural alerts in all of the 'positive' chemicals. About 25 per cent of the chemicals which were not classified as sensitizers were also found to contain structural alerts; these chemicals tended to be the ones containing ionic or polar groups and/or with large molecular weights, properties leading to lower skin permeability (Barratt and Basketter, 1994). Therefore, the great majority (60–70 per cent) of those chemicals in the database which contain a structural alert are regarded as having sufficiently high skin permeability to be classified as sensitizers. Thus, even on the conservative estimate that only 50 per cent of these chemicals could penetrate the skin to a sufficient extent, around one-third of all of the chemicals could be classified as skin sensitizers without any recourse to animal testing. It should be noted that this proportion of chemicals classifying as skin sensitizers agrees well with the experience of EU competent authorities (personal communication).

For chemicals which are not classified as sensitizers on the basis of their chemical and physical properties, the proposal is to test these in the LLNA according to the standard protocol (Kimber and Basketter, 1992). Since the LLNA uses just about half the number of animals required for OECD protocol guinea pig maximization tests (GPMT) and Buehler tests, animal usage would be cut by two-thirds if this proposed strategy was to be followed. An additional feature in favour of the LLNA from the animal welfare viewpoint is that it does not require the use of Freund's complete adjuvant, intradermal injections of test substance, fur removal, occlusive dressings or the use of restraint, all of which are features of the GPMT and/or the Buehler test. The proposed strategy presents an important opportunity for both substantial reduction and refinement of animal usage in a manner which will

Table 5.2 ECETOC dataset (ex Kimber *et al.*, 1995)

Chemical[1]	Sensitizer[2]	DEREK[3]	Skin penetration[4]	LLNA[5]
2,4-Dinitrochlorobenzene	+	+	high	+
Formaldehyde	+	+	high	+
Potassium dichromate	+	+	low	+
Isoeugenol	+	+	high	+
4-Ethoxymethylene-2-phenyl-2-oxazol-5-one	+	+	high	+
Paraphenylenediamine	+	+	moderate	+
Ethylenediamine	+	+	high	+
Cinnamic aldehyde	+	+	high	+
Kathon CG	+	+	high	+
Dowicil 200	+	+	moderate	+
Cobalt chloride	+	+	low	+
Nickel sulphate	+	+	low	−
Hexyl cinnamic aldehyde	+	+	high	+
Benzocaine	+	+	moderate	+/−
Mercaptobenzothiazole	+	+	high	+
Glutaraldehyde	+	+	high	+
Hydroxyethylacrylate	+	+	moderate	+
Penicillin G	+	+	moderate	+
Toluene diamine bismaleimide	+	+	moderate	+
Eugenol	+	+	high	+
Cocoamidopropylbetaine	+	−	low	+
Citral	+	+	high	+
Ethylene glycol dimethacrylate	+	+	high	+
Hydroxycitronellal	+	+	moderate	+
Diphenylthiourea	+	+	moderate	+
Methyl salicylate	−	−	high	−
Sodium dodecyl sulphate	−	−	low	+/−
p-Aminobenzoic acid	−	+	low	−
Diethylphthalate	−	−	high	
2-Hydroxypropyl methacrylate	−	+	moderate	−
Glycerol	−	−	low	
Zinc sulphate	−	−	low	
Isopropanol	−	−	moderate	
Lead acetate	−	−	low	
Olive oil	−	−	low	−
Tartaric acid	−	−	moderate	
Dimethyl formamide	−	−	high	−

[1]The list of chemicals is from the European Centre for Ecotoxicology and Toxicology of Chemicals (ECETOC) (Kimber *et al.*, 1995).
[2]Classification based on EU criteria.
[3]DEREK expert system assessment of the presence of a structural alert for skin sensitization.
[4]Expert view on likelihood of skin penetration, including evaluation of log *P* and molecular volume by computation.
[5]Result of testing in the LLNA. Data taken from previous publications (Kimber *et al.*, 1994; Basketter *et al.*, 1994).

not compromise the existing standard of classification and labelling of skin sensitization hazard in the EU (Basketter *et al.*, 1995).

It is important to demonstrate that this strategy can work successfully with datasets of chemicals which either do or do not classify as skin sensitisers, for example, an assessment of the list of positive and negative substances specifically proposed by the European Centre for Ecotoxicology and Toxicology of Chemicals (ECETOC) for the purposes of novel test evaluation (Kimber *et al.*, 1995). Table 5.2 shows their categorization as skin sensitizers, the assessment by the DEREK rulebase, a broad assessment of their skin penetration characteristics and the LLNA result. Of the 25 sensitizing chemicals, all but one are identified by the DEREK rulebase as containing structural alerts for skin sensitization. That chemical, cocoamidopropyl-betaine, has recently been shown to be a sensitizer due to the presence of 3-dimethylaminopropylamine (Angelini *et al.*, 1995), a chemical used in the manufacture, and is correctly identified by the LLNA. Of the 12 chemicals not classified in the EU as skin sensitizers, only two were identified by the DEREK rulebase as containing structural alerts. One of these chemicals, *p*-aminobenzoic acid, is unlikely to be a significant skin sensitizer due to its poor ability to penetrate skin (see above); this is confirmed by the negative LLNA. Hydroxypropyl methacrylate met DEREK criteria for skin sensitization and was also assessed to be 'moderate' for skin penetration and thus might be judged to be a false positive. The remaining 10 chemicals did not contain structural alerts for skin sensitization and with the exception of SLS, which at times is slightly positive in the LLNA (Kimber and Basketter, 1992; Basketter *et al.*, 1994), were all negative in the LLNA assay.

Conclusion

The strategic approach described above permits the correct identification of chemicals which should be classified as skin sensitizers. Furthermore this correct identification is not achieved by significant over-classification of non-sensitizers. The approach has considerable merit on animal welfare grounds and is both rapid and highly cost effective. Thus, whilst it does not seek to change existing regulatory thresholds, it does offer a real opportunity for an improvement in the hazard identification process since the strategy is based on the fundamental mechanistic processes of skin sensitization. The evidence available strongly suggests that this strategy could be implemented now without compromising human safety. The value of this strategic approach will be demonstrated further in subsequent publications.

Acknowledgements

The authors wish to thank all of their colleagues, too numerous to name individually, who have collaborated in different aspects of this work over a number of years.

References

ANGELINI, G., FOTI, C., RIGANO, L. and VENA, G.A. 1995, 3-Dimethylaminopropylamine: a key substance in contact allergy to cocamidopropylbetaine? *Contact Dermatitis*, **32**, 96–9.

ASHBY, J., HILTON, J., DEARMAN, R.J., CALLANDER, R.D. and KIMBER, I. 1993, Mechanistic relationship among mutagenicity, skin sensitization and skin carcinogenicity, *Environmental Health Perspectives*, **101**, 62–7.

BARRATT, M.D. 1995, Quantitative structure activity relationships for skin permeability, *Toxicology in Vitro*, **9**, 27–37.

BARRATT, M.D. and BASKETTER, D.A. 1992, Possible origin of the skin sensitization potential of isoeugenol and related compounds. (I) Preliminary studies of potential reaction mechanisms, *Contact Dermatitis*, **27**, 98–104.

1994, Structure-activity relationships for skin sensitization: an expert system. In: *In Vitro Toxicology*. A. Rougier, A.M. Goldberg and H.I. Maibach (eds.), Mary Ann Liebert, Inc., New York, pp. 293–301.

BARRATT, M.D., BASKETTER, D.A., CHAMBERLAIN, M., ADMANS, G.D. and LANGOWSKI, J.J. 1994a, An expert system rulebase for identifying contact allergens, *Toxicology in Vitro*, **8**, 1053–60.

BARRATT, M.D., BASKETTER, D.A. and ROBERTS, D.W. 1994b, Skin sensitization structure activity relationships for phenyl benzoates, *Toxicology in Vitro*, **8**, 823–6.

BASKETTER, D. 1992, Skin sensitization to cinnamic alcohol: The role of skin metabolism, *Acta Dermatologica Venereologica*, **72**, 264–5.

BASKETTER, D.A. and ROBERTS, D.W. 1990, A quantitative structure activity/dose relationship for contact allergic potential of alkyl group transfer agents, *Toxicology in Vitro*, **4**, 686–7.

BASKETTER, D.A., ROBERTS, D.W., CRONIN, M. and SCHOLES, E.W. 1992, The value of the local lymph node assay in quantitative structure activity investigations, *Contact Dermatitis*, **27**, 137–42.

BASKETTER, D.A., SCHOLES, E.W. and KIMBER, I. 1994, Performance of the local lymph node assay with chemicals found identified as contact allergens in the human maximisation test. *Food and Chemical Toxicology*, **32**, 543–7.

BASKETTER, D.A., SCHOLES, E.W., CHAMBERLAIN, M. and BARRATT, M.D. 1995, An alternative strategy to the use of guinea pigs for the identification of skin sensitization hazard, *Food and Chemical Toxicology*, **33**, in press.

BENEZRA, C. and DUCOMBS, G. 1987, Molecular aspects of allergic contact dermatitis to plants. Recent progress in phytodermatochemistry, *Dermatosen in Beruf und Umwelt*, **35**, 4–11.

BENEZRA, C. and EPSTEIN, W.L. 1986, Molecular recognition patterns of sesquiterpene lactones in costus-sensitive patients, *Contact Dermatitis*, **15**, 223–30.

BENEZRA, C., STAMPF, J-L., BARBIER, P. and DUCOMBS, G. 1985, Enantiospecificity in allergic contact dermatitis. A review and new results in Frullania-sensitive patients, *Contact Dermatitis*, **13**, 110–4.

BERGMAN, H.H., BEIJERSBERGER, J.C.H., OVERGEEM, J.C. and SIJPESTEIJN, A.K. 1967, Isolation and identification of α-methylene butyrolactone: a fungitoxic substance from tulips, *Recueil Travail Chimie Pays-Bas*, **86**, 709–13.

CHASE, M.W. 1947, Sensitization of animals with simple chemical compounds. X. Antibodies inducing immediate-type skin reactions, *Journal of Experimental*

Medicine, **86**, 480–514.

CRONIN, M.T.D. and BASKETTER, D.A. 1994, Multivariate QSAR analysis of a skin sensitization database, *SAR and QSAR in Environmental Research*, **2**, 159–79.

DAVIES, M.S., MILE, B., ROWLANDS, C.C. and BARRATT, M.D. 1995, Oxidation of 4-methylcatechol by dioxygen studied by ESR spectroscopy. The different regioselectivity of OH⁻ and MeO⁻ nucleophilic attack and kinetic deuterium isotope effects, *Magnetic Resonance in Chemistry*, **33**, 15–9.

DE GROOT, A.C., WEYLAND, J.W. and NATER, J.P. 1994, *Unwanted Effects of Cosmetics and Drugs used in Dermatology*. Elsevier, Amsterdam.

DUPUIS, G. 1979, Studies of poison ivy. In vitro lymphocyte transformation by urushiol protein conjugates, *British Journal of Dermatology*, **101**, 617–24.

DUPUIS, G. and BENEZRA, C. 1982, *Contact Dermatitis to Simple Chemicals: A Molecular Approach*. Marcel Dekker, New York.

EEC 1983, EEC Commission Directive of 29 July 1983 adapting to technical progress for the fifth time Directive 67/548/EEC on the approximation of laws, regulations and administrative provisions relating to the classification, packaging and labelling of dangerous substances. (Annex V). *Official Journal of the European Communities*, **L257**, 1.

EU 1993, Council Directive 92/32/EEC. 7th Amendment to Directive 67/548/EEC. *Official Journal of the European Communities 35*, **L154**.

EVANS, J.C., JACKSON, S.K., ROWLANDS, C.C. and BARRATT, M.D. 1985, An electron spin resonance study of radicals from chloramine-T. Part 1; Spin trapping of radicals produced in acid media, *Tetrahedron*, **41**, 5191–94.

1986, Covalent binding of human serum albumin and ovalbumin by chloramine-T and chemical modification of the proteins, *Analytica Chimica Acta*, **186**, 319–23.

FRANOT, C., ROBERTS, D.W., SMITH, R.G., BASKETTER, D.A., BENEZRA, C. and LEPOITTEVIN, J-P. 1994a, Structure activity relationships for contact allergenic potential of γ,γ-dimethyl-γ-butyrolactone derivatives. 1. Synthesis and electrophilic reactivity studies of α-(ω-substituted-alkyl)-γ,γ-dimethyl-γ-butyrolactones and correlation of skin sensitization potential and cross-sensitization patterns with structure, *Chemical Research in Toxicology*, **7**, 297–306.

FRANOT, C., ROBERTS, D.W., BASKETTER, D.A., BENEZRA, C. and LEPOITTEVIN, J-P. 1994b, Structure activity relationships for contact allergenic potential of γ,γ-dimethyl,l-γ-butyrolactone derivatives. 2. Quantitative structure-skin sensitization relationship for α-(ω-substituted-alkyl)-γ,γ-dimethyl-γ-butyrolactones, *Chemical Research in Toxicology*, **7**, 307–12.

FRANOT, C., BENEZRA, C. and LEPOITTEVIN, J-P. 1993, Synthesis and interaction studies of 13C labelled lactone derivatives with a model protein using 13C NMR, *Bioorganic and Medicinal Chemistry*, **1**, 389–97.

FRIEDMAN, P.S. and MOSS, C. 1985, Quantification of contact hypersensitivity in man. In: *Models in Dermatology*, Vol. 2, H.I. Maibach and N. Lowe (eds.), Karger, Basel, pp. 275–81.

FLYNN, G.L. 1990, Physicochemical determinants of skin absorption. In: *Principles of Route-to-Route Extrapolation for Risk Assessment*, T.R. Gerrity and C.J. Henry (eds.), Elsevier Science Publishing Co., Inc., New York, pp. 93–127.

GÄFVERT, E., SHAO, L.P., KARLBERG, A-T., NILSSON, U. and NILSSON, J.L.G. 1994, Contact allergy to resin hydroperoxides. Hapten binding via free radicals and epoxides, *Chemical Research in Toxicology*, **7**, 260–6.

GOODWIN, B.F.J., CREVEL, R.W.R. and JOHNSON, A.W. 1981, A comparison of three guinea pig sensitization procedures for the detection of 19 reported human contact sensitizers, *Contact Dermatitis*, **7**, 248–58.

GOODWIN, B.F.J. and JOHNSON, A.W. 1985, Single injection adjuvant test. In: *Current Problems in Dermatology*, Vol. 14, Anderson, K.E. and Maibach, H.I. (eds.), pp. 201–7.

GUILLOT, J.P., GONNET, J-F., CLEMENT, C. and FACCINI, J.M. 1983, Comparative study of methods chosen by the Association Française de Normalisation (AFNOR) for evaluating sensitization potential in the albino guinea pig, *Food and Chemical Toxicology*, **21**, 795–805.

HELLERSTROM, S., THYRESSON N., BLOHM, S-G. and WIDMARK, G. 1955, On the nature of the eczematogenic component of oxidised Δ^3-carene, *Journal of Investigative Dermatology*, **24**, 21–224.

HINZ, R.S., LORENCE, C.R., HODSON, C.D., HANSCH, C., HALL, L.L. and GUY, R.H. 1991, Percutaneous penetration of para-substituted phenols in vitro, *Fundamental and Applied Toxicology*, **17**, 575–83.

HOTCHKISS, S.A.M. 1992, Skin as a xenobiotic metabolizing organ. In: *Progress in Drug Metabolism*, Vol. 13, G.G. Gibson (ed.), Taylor and Francis, London, pp. 217–67.

HOTCHKISS, S.A.M. 1995, Cutaneous toxicity. Kinetic and metabolic determinants, *Toxicology and Ecotoxicology News*, **2**, 10–18.

KANIWA, M-A., MOMMA, J., IKARASHI, Y., KOJIMA, S., NAKAMURA, A., NAKAJI, Y., KUROKAWA, Y., KANTOH, H. and ITOH, M. 1992, A method for identifying causative chemicals of allergic contact dermatitis using a combination of chemical analysis and patch testing in patients and animal groups: Application to a case of rubber boot dermatitis, *Contact Dermatitis*, **27**, 166–73.

KAO, J. and CARVER, M.P. 1990, Cutaneous metabolism of xenobiotics, *Drug Metabolism Reviews*, **22**, 363–410.

KARLBERG, A-T., MAGNUSSON, K. and NILSSON, U. 1992, Air oxidation of d-limonene – the citrus solvent – creates potent allergens, *Contact Dermatitis*, **26**, 332–40.

KARLBERG, A-T. 1991, Air oxidation increases the allergic potential of Tall Oil Rosin. Colophony contact allergens also identified in Tall Oil Rosin, *American Journal of Contact Dermatitis*, **2**, 43–9.

KIMBER, I. and BASKETTER, D.A. 1992, The murine local lymph node assay; collaborative studies and new directions: A commentary, *Food and Chemical Toxicology*, **30**, 165–9.

KIMBER, I., DEARMAN, R.J., SCHOLES, E.W. and BASKETTER, D.A. 1994, The local lymph node assay: developments and applications, *Toxicology*, **93**, 13–31.

KIMBER, I., BASKETTER, D.A., BRIATICO-VANGOSA, G., COOKMAN, G., EVANS, P., LOVELESS, S. and PAULUHN, J. 1995, ms in prep.

KLIGMAN, A.M. 1966, The identification of contact allergens by human assay. III. The maximization test: a procedure for screening and rating contact sensitizers, *Journal of Investigative Dermatology*, **47**, 393–409.

LANDSTEINER, K. and JACOBS, J.L. 1936, Studies on the sensitization of animals with simple chemicals III, *Journal of Experimental Medicine*, **64**, 625–39.

LEPOITTEVIN, J-P. and KARLBERG, A-T. 1994, Interaction of allergic hydroperoxides with proteins, *Chemical Research in Toxicology*, **7**, 130–3.

LIBERATO, D.J., BYERS, V., DENNICK, R.G. and CASTAGNOLI, N. Jr. 1981, Regiospecific attack of nitrogen and sulphur nucleophiles on quinones derived from poison oak/ivy catechols (urushiols) and analogues as models for urushiol-protein conjugate formation, *Journal of Medicinal Chemistry*, **24**, 28–33.

MAGEE, P.S., HOSTYNEK, J.J. and MAIBACH, H.I. 1994, A classification model for allergic contact dermatitis, *Quantitative Structure – Activity Relationships*, **13**, 22–33.

MARCHANT, B., BARBIER, P., DUCOMBS, G., FOUSSEREAU, J., MARTIN, P. and BENEZRA, C. 1982, Allergic contact dermatitis to various salols (phenyl salicylates). A structure activity relationship study in man and in animal (guinea pig), *Archives of Dermatological Research*, **272**, 61–6.

MARTIN, R.J., DENYER, S.P. and HADGRAFT, J. 1987, Skin metabolism of topically applied compounds, *International Journal of Pharmaceutics*, **39**, 23–32.

MAYER, R.L. 1954, Group sensitization to compounds of quinone structure and its biochemical basis. Role of these substances in cancer, *Progress in Allergy*, **4**, 79–172.

MOTTEN, A.G., CHIGNELL, C.F. and MASON, R.P. 1983, Spectroscopic studies of cutaneous photosensitizing agents – VI. Identification of the free radicals generated during the photolysis of musk ambrette, musk xylene and musk ketone, *Photochemistry and Photobiology*, **5**, 365–9.

PAPAGEORGIOU, C., CORBET, J-C., MENEZES-BRANDAO, F., PECEGUEIRO, M. and BENEZRA, C. 1983, Allergic contact dermatitis to garlic (*Allium sativum L.*). Identification of the allergens: The role of mono-, di- and trisulfides present in garlic, *Archives of Dermatological Research*, **275**, 229–34.

PENDLINGTON, R.U. and BARRATT, M.D. 1990, The molecular basis of photocontact allergy, *International Journal of Cosmetic Science*, **12**, 91–103.

POTTS, R.O. and GUY, R., 1992, Predicting skin permeability, *Pharmaceutical Research*, **9**, 663–9.

RAO, K.S. BETSO, J.E. and OHLSON, K.J. 1981, A collection of guinea pig sensitization test results grouped by chemical class, *Drug and Chemical Toxicology*, **4**, 331–51.

ROBERTS, D.W. 1987, Structure activity relationship for skin sensitization potential of diacrylates and dimethacrylates, *Contact Dermatitis*, **17**, 281–9.

ROBERTS, D.W. and BASKETTER, D.A. 1990, A quantitative structure activity/dose response relationship for contact allergic potential of alkyl group transfer agents, *Contact Dermatitis*, **23**, 331–5.

ROBERTS, D.W. and WILLIAMS, D.L. 1992, The derivation of quantitative correlations between skin sensitization and physicochemical parameters for alkylating agents, and their application to experimental data for sultones, *Journal of Theoretical Biology*, **99**, 807–25.

1983, Sultones as by-products in anionic surfactants, *Tenside Detergents*, **20**, 109–11.

SANDERSON, D.M. and EARNSHAW, C.G. 1991, Computer prediction of possible toxic action from chemical structure; The DEREK system, *Human and Experimental Toxicology*, **10**, 261–73.

SCHMIDT, R.J., KHAN, L. and CHUNG, L.Y. 1990, Are free radicals and not quinones the haptenic species derived from urushiols and other contact allergenic mono- and dihydric alkylbenzenes? The significance of NADH, glutathione and redox cycling in the skin, *Archives of Dermatological Research*, **282**, 56–64.

SUZUKI, T. 1991, Development of an automated system for both partition coefficient and aqueous solubility, *Journal of Computer-Aided Molecular Design*, **5**, 149–66.

VECCHINI, F., MACE, K., MAGDALOU, J., MAHE, Y., BERNARD, B.A. and SHROOT, B. 1995, Constitutive and inducible expression of drug metabolising enzymes in cultured human keratinocytes, *British Journal of Dermatology*, **132**, 14–21.

6

Regulatory Aspects of Contact Hypersensitivity

P. EVANS

Health and Safety Executive, Bootle

Introduction

It is probably fair to say that the processes of governmental regulatory authorities have not always been held in high regard by scientists working in industry. Regulators have sometimes been considered to be 'box-tickers' that used a mystifying assortment of legislative directives, amendments, annexes and adaptations to guide their decisions and justify their demands. This situation does not advance what is essentially a common cause approached from different perspectives. After all, regulating means permitting as well as restricting – it is about finding the right balance. Similarly, industry has shared responsibility with, for example, the Health and Safety Executive (HSE) in its mission 'to ensure that risks to people's health and safety from work are properly controlled'.

Times are changing and increasingly regulatory positions in relation to toxicology must be scientifically sound and fully explained. Contact hypersensitivity has probably generated more discussion, regarding both the validity of test protocols and the interpretation of test results for classification purposes, than any other single toxicological endpoint in regulatory programmes for industrial chemicals. The overriding need of the regulatory authority is to be convinced that the test performed on a particular chemical has been done stringently, so that there is a minimal likelihood that a false-negative or, indeed, a false-positive result has been obtained. Against this background, the present chapter aims to address some of the issues that engage regulatory toxicologists when they assess reports of contact hypersensitivity studies conducted for these programmes. It is hoped that it will be of value to those who need to submit contact hypersensitivity tests for regulatory appraisal.

The Guidance Available

Reports of contact hypersensitivity studies are submitted to regulatory authorities in association with, for example, European Union (EU) programmes concerned with the notification, classification and labelling and risk assessment of 'new' and 'existing' chemicals. Approved test methods for use in these programmes have been published by the EU, and are commonly known as the Annex V methods. This is because they are presented as the fifth technical annex to the Dangerous Substances Directive (EEC, 1967). The first Annex V method for contact hypersensitivity (EEC, 1984) was based on the existing guideline for skin sensitization produced by the competent international body for testing methods, the Organisation for Economic Co-operation and Development (OECD, 1981). In 1989–1990, the Annex V method was revised to take into account technical progress, but due to unforeseen delays the updated method was not finally published until the end of 1992. In the meantime, the OECD was also working on a revised guideline which, although published (OECD, 1992) at about the same time as the Annex V method, was actually based on more recent scientific and regulatory thinking. In effect, it 'leap-frogged' over the Annex V method to become the authoritative source of regulatory guidance on the conduct of contact hypersensitivity studies. Clearly though, use of the Annex V method will still ensure regulatory compliance.

Guidance on the standardized performance of the guinea pig maximization test has recently been provided by a German regulatory authority (Schlede and Eppler, 1995). Also, sensible proposals for updating this assay have been made, in the light of experience of its use over many years (Kligman and Basketter, 1995).

Criteria to be applied to the results of contact hypersensitivity studies, in order to derive the appropriate classification and labelling for the test substance, are available in Annex VI to the Dangerous Substances Directive, which is often referred to as the 'labelling guide' (EEC, 1993).

Acceptable Types of Test

The original Annex V method for contact hypersensitivity described the conduct of the guinea pig maximization test in some detail, referring to it as the preferred (reference) method. An appendix tabulated key details of six other guinea pig tests, namely the Draize, Freund's complete adjuvant, Maurer optimization, Buehler, open epicutaneous and split adjuvant assays, but without giving any encouragement for their use. The OECD guideline on which this version of Annex V was based apparently considered all seven of these tests equally acceptable. It gave a common, general description of the conduct of a study, together with individual details for each in a table. In an annex it also provided guidance on a footpad technique, which was not considered to be widely used.

By comparison, the updated Annex V method gives specific guidance on the maximization test (the preferred adjuvant method) and the Buehler test (the preferred non-adjuvant method). It considers that in general adjuvant tests are preferred over non-adjuvant tests, because of their likely greater sensitivity and hence ability to predict an effect in humans. Although it is recognized that for some substances a non-adjuvant test may be more appropriate, it is an explicit requirement that 'scientific justification should be given when the Buehler test is used'.

The usual reasons for not conducting a maximization test are associated with injection of the test substance at the first stage of induction. The substance may be too viscous for injection, or may not dissolve or disperse in the usual vehicles. However, if a range of solvents is tried, generally one can be found that permits injection of the test substance. Another potential problem with intradermal injection arises if the substance is corrosive or strongly irritant, so that necrotic and ulcerative reactions occur at the injection site. These effects may be exacerbated by the simultaneous administration of adjuvant. In general, however, careful selection of the intradermal induction concentration (using data obtained in the preliminary 'sighting' study) should allow these severe reactions to be avoided. Thus, it seems that it is technically possible to perform a maximization test for the great majority of substances, and indeed more than 90 per cent of the contact hypersensitivity tests on new substances submitted to the EU are maximization tests (Schlede and Eppler, 1995). However, it must be recognized that testing for contact hypersensitivity is not as yet globally harmonized, so that reports of tests other than maximization studies (for example, Buehler tests carried out in N. America) are occasionally received by EU regulatory authorities. In the interests of animal welfare, it is appropriate that the results of these tests are properly assessed and utilized if possible, and that the study is not rejected unless there are overriding scientific reasons.

In the updated Annex V method no tests other than the maximization and the Buehler are mentioned by name, although it is stated that 'other methods may be used provided that they are well-validated and scientific justification is given'. Clearly this statement begs a number of questions, and these will be addressed below when the choice of an appropriate positive control substance is discussed.

The updated OECD guideline introduces the possibility of using positive results obtained with mice (using the mouse ear swelling test or the local lymph node assay) to identify a substance as a potential skin sensitizer, and thus avoid the need to test in guinea pigs. However, if a negative result is obtained in the mouse assay, this is not currently acceptable for classification purposes, and a guinea pig test must be conducted subsequently in order to confirm that the substance is not a sensitizer. The challenge currently facing the mouse assays is to achieve full validation, so that negative findings (which do not lead to classification and labelling) also become acceptable to regulatory authorities.

Showing consistency with the updated Annex V method, the updated OECD guideline describes both the maximization and Buehler tests in detail. These are clearly the recommended methods, although it is recognized that other (unspecified) assays may be used when appropriate.

Although no method even approaching regulatory status is currently available, the development of an *in vitro* screen for skin sensitization is a goal that remains desirable and in theory appears reasonable, given that individual components of the sensitization reaction (such as the ability to penetrate skin and to bind to protein) can be assessed using *in vitro* techniques.

Positive Control Substances

Although it is not necessary to run concurrent positive controls with every contact hypersensitivity test, the sensitivity and reliability of the method being used should be assessed regularly using known sensitizers. The original OECD guideline was vague in this respect, recommending 'periodic use of a positive control substance with an acceptable level of response'. The original Annex V method was only slightly more helpful, calling for checking at six-monthly intervals using 'known strong and moderate sensitizers' and for a 'satisfactory number of positive responses'.

The revised guidance, however, is much more explicit. Unfortunately, the updated Annex V method is potentially confusing in that although in its introduction it calls for checking sensitivity using a known mild-to-moderate sensitizer, it later recommends as 'reference substances' para-phenylenediamine, 2,4-dinitrochlorobenzene, potassium dichromate, neomycin sulphate and nickel sulphate which have been 'diluted as necessary'. The first three of these substances are generally considered to be strong sensitizers. Given this apparent contradiction, the updated OECD guideline provides clearer guidance. It indicates that the reliability check should use substances which are known to have mild-to-moderate skin sensitizing properties, and should obtain a response in at least 30 per cent of the animals in an adjuvant test or at least 15 per cent in a non-adjuvant test. The preferred substances are listed as hexylcinnamic aldehyde, mercaptobenzothiazole and benzocaine, although other positive control substances meeting the same criteria are allowed with 'adequate justification'.

The introduction of the use of mild-to-moderate sensitizers to define the sensitivity of the assay system used has important implications for the selection of the test method in the first place. If the method consistently gives adequate sensitization response rates with one or more of the OECD-recommended positive control substances, it would not be reasonable to reject that method on the grounds that it lacks sensitivity. This is obviously more likely to be relevant to methods other than the maximization test, and would apply, for example, to the 'other methods' referred to in the updated Annex V guidance as requiring validation and scientific justification. Conversely, an assay previously acceptable to a regulatory authority because it responded well to a strong sensitizer such as dinitrochlorobenzene, but now found to give an inadequate sensitization response with mild-to-moderate sensitizers, would require refinement to increase its sensitivity.

Numbers of Animals

In the earlier guidance for the maximization test, groups of 20 treated and 10 control guinea pigs were stipulated in Annex V (EEC, 1984), and groups of 20–25 recommended in each case in the OECD guideline (OECD, 1981). More recently, however, there have been demonstrations of the feasibility of using only 10 treated and 5 control animals, but obtaining the same conclusions regarding the need to classify the substance as a skin sensitizer as when the full '20 and 10' Annex V method is followed (Hofmann *et al.*, 1987; Shillaker *et al.*, 1989). The EU scheme requires classification of a substance as a skin sensitizer when it causes a response in at least 30 per cent of the animals in an adjuvant test (EEC, 1993).

In the light of this development, the updated versions of both sets of guidance now state that a minimum of 10 animals is used for the treated group and at least five for the control group. Unfortunately, the addition of qualifying statements in each case has blunted their impact in reducing the numbers of animals used in contact hypersensitivity tests. Also, slight differences in the wording of these statements have led to some confusion. The Annex V method has 'when it is not possible to conclude definitively that the test substance is or is not a sensitizer, testing in additional animals to give a total of at least 20 test and 10 control animals is recommended'. The OECD wording is similar, but omits 'definitively' and 'or is not', and adds 'strongly' before 'recommended'.

The practical significance of these differences is not great, although a literal interpretation has a response of 0/10 being acceptable evidence for lack of sensitizing potential, without the need for further testing, according to the EU scheme but not according to the OECD guidance. More importantly, however, the qualifications mean that since a significant proportion of '10 and 5' tests (i.e. those with 0, 1 or 2 /10 test guinea pigs showing sensitization reactions under the OECD guideline, those with one or two positive animals according to Annex V) will need to be repeated to bring them up to '20 and 10', it will in some cases appear more practical to conduct a '20 and 10' study from the outset. For animal welfare reasons, however, it is strongly recommended that a '10 and 5' study is initially performed, then repeated if necessary. In the event of a clear positive response (i.e. 3–10/10 sensitization reactions), or completely negative findings in this initial test, no further animals need to be tested. If the result of the initial test is equivocal in classification terms (i.e. there are 1 or 2/10 sensitized guinea pigs in the test group), the test will need to be repeated. However, there will be a benefit in that over a period of time it will become possible to assess the value of this repetition in determining the eventual classifications of the test substances. For the Buehler test, the original versions of both Annex V and the OECD guideline indicated 10–20 guinea pigs for both test and control groups. The updated versions agree in requiring a minimum of 20 animals in the treated group and at least 10 in the control group.

Induction and Challenge Concentrations

These concentrations should be determined from the findings of preliminary tests using two or three guinea pigs. For a maximization study, it may be appropriate to use adjuvant-treated animals for this 'sighting' test. The concentrations chosen for each stage of induction should be well-tolerated systemically, and produce some evidence of skin irritation (EEC, 1992). The OECD guideline defines these concentrations as the highest to cause mild-to-moderate skin irritation (OECD, 1992). In maximizing the induction conditions, the assay should not necessarily be limited by the maximum concentrations (5 per cent intradermally, 25 per cent topically) originally prescribed for the assay (Magnusson and Kligman, 1969). However, a contrary view on this has been given (Schlede and Eppler, 1995). Recently, a good case has been made that control animals ought to be similarly exposed at induction to an irritant substance (e.g. sodium lauryl sulphate) to mimic the irritation produced by the test substance (Kligman and Basketter, 1995). Otherwise, a hyperirritable state induced in test animals but not control animals might lead to false-positive 'sensitization' reactions at challenge.

For the Buehler test, according to Annex V, the induction concentration should be the 'highest level that can be well tolerated systemically and which, for irritant substances, produces mild to moderate irritation in the majority of the test animals' (EEC, 1992). The OECD guideline states that the induction concentration should be the 'highest to cause mild irritation' (OECD, 1992).

The challenge concentration chosen for both maximization and Buehler tests should be the highest that produces no skin irritation (EEC, 1992; OECD, 1992). If the test substance is not irritant, the concentration could therefore be 100 per cent for a liquid. For a solid, the maximum concentration achievable would depend on its physicochemical properties, particularly its solubility in a suitable vehicle. For the maximization test, the maximum challenge concentration of 25 per cent advocated by Magnusson and Kligman (1969) does not necessarily apply.

Grading the Skin Reactions Found at Challenge

The Annex V method gives no guidance, but the updated OECD guideline introduced a grading scale based on that used by the originators of the maximization test (Magnusson and Kligman, 1969). This can be applied to skin reactions obtained at challenge in the Buehler as well as in maximization tests. The scale rises from 0 (no visible change), through 1 (discrete or patchy erythema) and 2 (moderate and confluent erythema) up to 3 (intense erythema and swelling). Some testing laboratories also record a minimal reaction, coming between 0 and 1 on this scale. This reaction is often designated '+/−' and may be described as 'red spots'.

Interpretation of Results for Classification Purposes

According to the EU classification scheme, if a substance produces sensitization reactions in 30 per cent or more of the guinea pigs tested in an adjuvant assay, or 15 per cent or more in a non-adjuvant assay, it will normally be classified as 'sensitizing' and the associated phrase R43 ('May cause sensitization by skin contact') will appear on the label of its package (EEC, 1993). When no skin reactions are seen in the control guinea pigs, the interpretation of the results for classification purposes is straightforward when clear-cut skin reactions, unequivocally indicative of sensitization, are obtained in the test animals at challenge. Even when the reactions in the test animals are of minimal grade (e.g. 'red spots'), if they are absent in the controls the current regulatory position is that they should be taken as evidence for sensitization (Schlede and Eppler, 1995). Recently, however, a re-evaluation of experience with the maximization test has concluded that weak challenge reactions may be evidence of either sensitization or irritation, so that false-positive results are possible (Kligman and Basketter, 1995). The mechanism proposed for these false-positive irritant reactions is that irritating induction doses of test substance cause a general state of hyperreactivity in the test animals. To distinguish between sensitization and false-positive irritation reactions obtained at challenge, it is therefore advisable to perform a second challenge after 1–3 weeks. True hypersensitivity reactions normally persist over this period (and often for much longer), while nonspecific irritation reactions tend to decrease or disappear, and rapid fading of a challenge reaction would also suggest irritation rather than sensitization (Kligman and Basketter, 1995).

Further uncertainty over interpretation of challenge reactions can arise when effects are also seen in the control animals. Since these must be irritant effects, they may cast doubt on the nature of the reactions apparent in the test animals, particularly if they are of the same grade. In this situation, one approach is to consider as evidence for sensitization only skin reactions in test animals that are of a higher grade than the maximum observed in any of the control animals. Thus an assay in which 8/20 test guinea pigs showed grade 2 and 12/20 grade 1 reactions would lead to classification of the test substance as a skin sensitizer even if 10/10 control animals also gave grade 1 reactions. However, there are potential pitfalls to this approach. For example, 19/20 grade 1 reactions seen in the test group would be countered by just one similar reaction found among the controls, so that no classification would follow.

An alternative approach to defining the percentage of test animals showing hypersensitivity is to subtract from the percentage of test animals showing skin reactions the percentage of control animals giving these reactions at challenge. Thus if 10/20 test and 1/10 control animals gave grade 1 effects, the response taken to be sensitization ($50 - 10 = 40\%$) would be sufficient to classify. Similarly, if there were 2/20 grade 2 and 18/20 grade 1 reactions in the test group, and 8/10 grade 1 effects in the control group, the sensitization response ($10 + [90 - 80] = 20\%$) would be enough to classify in a non-adjuvant but not in an adjuvant test.

Overall, there is probably no single method of evaluating challenge results for classification purposes that is appropriate for all circumstances. The approach taken will largely depend on the scientific judgement of those conducting the study, and the regulator can do nothing more than appraise that judgement on a case-by-case basis.

Concluding Statement

The testing of chemicals to discover their potential to cause contact hypersensitivity is an area of toxicology that has suffered more than most from uncertainties regarding the requirements of regulatory authorities. In a sentence, the regulator seeks reassurance that the tests are conducted stringently. To this end, clear guidance is needed to explain how such stringency is to be achieved. Guidance produced by the OECD and the EU has been updated relatively recently; in many respects the OECD guideline is consistent with the EU test method, but there are some significant differences. Also, in some specific areas the updated guidance has already been overtaken by more recent scientific developments.

In this chapter, the guidance available for regulatory testing for contact hypersensitivity has been discussed, and any differences and developments highlighted, with particular emphasis on the aspects which have caused uncertainty in the recent past. It is hoped that this will help to prevent similar uncertainty in the future. In any event, regulatory toxicologists will continue to welcome discussion on all aspects of testing for contact hypersensitivity, with a view to resolving problems encountered in regulatory programmes.

Acknowledgements

I am grateful to colleagues in HSE's Toxicology Unit, particularly Steve Fairhurst for providing inspiration for the introduction and Derek James for helpful comments on the drafts.

References

EEC, 1967, Council Directive 67/548/EEC, *Official Journal of the European Communities*, **196**, 1.

1984, Annex to Commission Directive 84/449/EEC, *Official Journal of the European Communities*, **L251**, 113–7.

1992, Annex to Commission Directive 92/69/EEC, *Official Journal of the European Communities*, **L383A**, 131–9.

1993, Annex to Commission Directive 93/21/EEC, *Official Journal of the European Communities*, **L110A**, 45–86.

HOFMANN, T., DIEHL, K.H., LEIST, K.H. and WEIGAND, W., 1987, The feasibility of sensitization studies using fewer test animals, *Archives of Toxicology*, **60**, 470–1.

KLIGMAN, A.M. and BASKETTER, D.A., 1995, A critical commentary and updating of the guinea pig maximization test, *Contact Dermatitis*, **32**, 129–34.

MAGNUSSON, B. and KLIGMAN, A.M., 1969, The identification of contact allergens by animal assay. The guinea pig maximization test, *Journal of Investigative Dermatology*, **52**, 268–76.

OECD, 1981, Guidelines for Testing of Chemicals, No 406, Skin Sensitisation.

1992, Guidelines for Testing of Chemicals, No 406, Skin Sensitisation.

SCHLEDE, E. and EPPLER, R., 1995, Testing for skin sensitization according to the notification procedure for new chemicals: the Magnusson and Kligman test, *Contact Dermatitis*, **32**, 1–4.

SHILLAKER, R.O., BELL, G.B., HODGSON, J.T. and PADGHAM, M.D.J., 1989, Guinea pig maximisation test for skin sensitisation: the use of fewer test animals, *Archives of Toxicology*, **63**, 283–8.

7

Guinea Pig Predictive Tests

T. MAURER

Ciba-Geigy Ltd, Basel

Introduction

Predictive guinea pig tests for evaluation of the skin sensitizing effects of chemicals have existed for nearly 50 years. The Draize test (Draize *et al.*, 1944; Johnson and Goodwin, 1985), was included in the first guideline in 1959 (Draize, 1959). The test was designed to screen out potent sensitizers. Negative results with known human sensitizers, such as benzocaine, neomycin and nickel sulphate (Magnusson and Kligman, 1969) and the simulation of the regular routes of exposure in man were the main reasons for developing other protocols.

Official guidelines for the testing of sensitizing effects were published in 1981 by the OECD and in 1984 by the EEC. The OECD guideline listed seven methods without giving preference to a particular test. The EEC favoured the use of the maximization test. Both guidelines described the test in tabular form and many modifications of the original protocol were possible. Approximately 5 years ago a working group of the Federal Health Office in Germany started to discuss reasonable changes to the existing guidelines. A limited number of tests was proposed for a new guideline (two adjuvant tests, two non-adjuvant tests); special preference was given for the maximization protocol (Schlede *et al.*, 1989). From a survey, organized by ECETOC, in Europe and the USA, it was apparent that the maximization test is the most frequently used method in Europe but that the Buehler test was the most common in the USA. Therefore, ECETOC (1990) proposed that preference be given to these two tests. In May 1991 an OECD expert meeting was held in Paris to discuss skin sensitization testing. The major changes which were captured for a new guideline which was accepted by the council on July 17, 1992 (OECD, 1992) were: 1) The protocol of Magnusson and Kligman and that of Buehler are recommended. Both protocols are described in detail. 2) If there are special reasons, other protocols can be used. 3) New reference compounds for internal validation are recommended (hexyl cinnamic aldehyde, 2-mercaptobenzothiazole, benzocaine) which have been proven recently to be sensitizers in two laboratories (Basketter *et al.*, 1993). 4) If a positive result in an early screening of compounds has been obtained in a mouse test (mouse ear swelling test = MEST or local lymph node assay = LLNA), no additional guinea pig test is necessary for registration of a new chemical. In contrast, a negative result in a mouse test must be confirmed in a guinea pig test, because the threshold of sensitivity of the mouse tests is not yet fully known. The same two tests are included also in the new EEC guideline of 1992. However, mouse screening data are not accepted. The guidelines are discussed also in Chapter 6.

Reviews on official and in-house guinea pig methods are given in Maurer (1983) and Andersen and Maibach (1985). Table 7.1 summarizes the principles of various test methods, such as route of administration and number of treatments. A selection of tests is described below in more detail.

Non-Adjuvant Tests

Draize Test and Modifications

As already mentioned, the main advantage of the Draize test (Draize *et al.*, 1944; Draize, 1959) is the great amount of experience in use as a result of its early development. The disadvantages are the lack of full standardization and its insensitivity for moderate or weak sensitizers (Table 7.2). Modifications of the Draize test, such as an increase of test concentrations (Voss, 1958) or repetition of the induction procedure (Sharp, 1978) have been made, but without a substantial increase in the sensitivity of the method.

Buehler Test

The Buehler test (Buehler, 1965, 1994; Buehler and Griffith 1975; Robinson *et al.*, 1990) was developed to screen strong and moderate sensitizers prior to testing in man. According to Buehler (1965), the test is more sensitive than the intradermal method developed by Draize and, when properly performed, of comparable sensitivity to that of an adjuvant-type test (Robinson *et al.*, 1990). One of the advantages is that the route of application is similar to that encountered in human use. A major disadvantage of the test was that different protocols were in use and that low incidences of positive animals were obtained with some known sensitizers (Table 7.3). A standard protocol is described in the publication of Robinson *et al.* (1990) and in the new OECD guideline of 1992. The impression of a lower sensitivity

Table 7.1 Guinea pig sensitization protocols

	Induction treatment		Challenge treatment	
	Application	Frequency	Application	Frequency
Non-adjuvant tests				
Draize (1944)	i.d.	10×	i.d.	1×
Buehler (1965)	occl., 6 hrs	3×/week, 3 weeks	occl., 6 hrs	1×
Robinson (1990)	occl., 6 hrs	1×/week, 3 weeks	occl., 6 hrs	1×
OET (Klecak, 1977)	topical	20×	topical 2 challenges	1×
Adjuvant tests				
Maximization				
(Magnusson and Kligman, 1969)	i.d. occl. 48 hrs	1×, 1×	occl., 24 hrs	1×
Optimization				
(Maurer *et al.*, 1975)	i.d.	10×	i.d. occl.	1× 1×
Modified Maximization				
(Sato, 1985)	i.d. occl. 24 hrs +SLS	1× 4×	topical	1×
FCAT (Klecak, 1977)	i.d.	3×	topical	
SIAT (Goodwin, 1981)	i.d.	1×	occl., 6 hrs	1×
CCET (Tsuchiya, 1985)	i.d. occl., 24 hrs	1×; 4×	topical	1×
Modified Maximization				
(Maurer and Hess, 1989)	i.d. occl., 48 hrs	1× 1×	occl.	1× 1×
CA2 Test (Kashima, 1993b)	CY i.d. occl., 24 hrs	1× 2× 2×	topical	1×

i.d. = intradermal injection, topical = epidermal open application, occl. = epidermal occlusive application, CY = cyclophosphamide, SLS = sodium lauryl sulphate.

of the Buehler test compared with adjuvant tests may be due also to not having followed the protocol properly. Advice for the performance of the Buehler test is given in the publication of Buehler (1994). Critical parameters are: selection of vehicles, selection of the induction concentration and type of occlusion. The ability of the test to detect known allergens has also been improved using an occlusive application device, the Hill Top Chamber® (Polikandritou and Conine, 1985).

Table 7.2   Results obtained with the Draize protocol and modifications

Compound	Number of positive animals per group			
	Buehler (1965)	Magnusson (1969)	Klecak (1977)	Sharp (1978)
TCSA	0/10	2/25		
PPD	0/10			
Benzocaine	0/10	0/25		
Pot. dichr.	1/10	3/20		
Formaldehyde	1/10	1/20		
Cinn. ald.			+	+
Citral			+	−
Citronellal			−	−
Salicylates			−	−

TCSA = tetrachlorosalicylanilide, PPD = *p*-phenylene diamine, Pot. dichr. = potassium dichromate, Cinn. ald. = cinnamic aldehyde.

Table 7.3   Results obtained with the Buehler protocol

Compound	Number of positive animals per group		
	Buehler (1965, 1975)	Polikandritou (1985)	
		HTC	WP
TCSA	8/10		
PPD	10/10	9/10	5/10
Benzocaine	2/10		
Pot. dichr.	1/10	6/10	3/10
Formaldehyde	3/10		
Neomycin		7/10	2/10
CPY	0/20		

TCSA = tetrachlorosalicylanilide, PPD = *p*-phenylene diamine, Pot. dichr. = potassium dichromate, CPY = 1-(3-chlorophenyl)-3-(4-chlorophenyl)-2-pyrazoline, HTC = Hill Top Chamber®, WP = webril patch.

Open Epidermal Tests

An open epidermal test was introduced in 1962 by Weirich. The method, which included 15 topical treatments during induction, was developed primarily for the screening of strong sensitizers before testing in man. An ear flank test was published by Stevens in 1967. In 1977, Klecak *et al.* described the open epidermal test (OET) which includes 20 epidermal open

Table 7.4 Results obtained with the maximization protocol

| Compound | Number of positive animals per group | | |
| | Magnusson and Kligman (1969) | Maurer and Hess (1989) | |
		Standard protocol	Modified protocol
TCSA	18/25		
Benzocaine	7/25	6/10	5/10
Pot. dichr.	18/24		8/10
Formaldehyde	10/20	9/10	7/10
Neomycin	18/25		
DNCB		20/20	20/20
PPD		20/20	10/10
CPY		20/20	10/10

TCSA = tetrachlorosalicylanilide, Pot. dichr. = potassium dichromate, DNCB = dinitrochlorobenzene, CPY = pyrazoline derivate.

applications for induction and single open treatments for two separate challenges. This is the only test using different concentrations of the test compound for induction and challenge. According to Klecak *et al.* (1977) it is possible to define the minimal sensitizing and eliciting concentration for each compound. Most experience with the test has been gained testing fragrances. Consequently, its reliability for the prediction of the sensitizing potential of industrial chemicals is not well known. Comparison with other tests is very difficult because no incidences of positive animals are given in the publications and no threshold of positive animals per group is provided for a positive result.

Adjuvant Tests

Maximization Test

The major steps introduced to enhance the sensitivity of the guinea pig methods in the maximization test of Magnusson and Kligman (1969) were: 1) injections of Freund's complete adjuvant (FCA) during the induction phase, 2) the use of maximal tolerated concentrations, 3) irritation of the application site before the epidermal induction treatment for chemicals which are not themselves irritant.

The sensitivity of the test is high and all known sensitizers which are negative in the Draize test are positive in the maximization test (Table 7.4). The major increase of sensitivity with the maximization protocol derives from the adjuvant injections. The additional role of the sodium lauryl sulphate

Table 7.5 Results obtained with the optimization protocol

Compound	Incidence of positive animals Maurer (1985)	
	i.d. chall.	epid. chall.
Dinitrochlorobenzene	20/20	20/20
Formaldehyde	20/20	10/20
Tetrachlorosalicylanilide	11/20	19/19
p-Phenylene diamine	20/20	13/20
Potassium dichromate	19/20	13/20
Pyrazoline derivate (CPY)	19/20	17/20
Neomycin	11/20	2/20
Methyl paraben	3/20	4/20
Propyl paraben	10/20	0/20
Phenoxy ethanol	1/20	0/20
	13/20*	0/20
Phenyl propanol	2/20	0/20
	14/20*	3/20

i.d. chall. = intradermal challenge, epid. chall. = epidermal occlusive challenge. * = 2 per cent induction concentration.

(SLS) pretreatment, which should enhance skin penetration, is not clear. Wilhelm *et al.* (1991) tested the penetration of four pharmaceuticals of diverse physicochemical properties in hairless guinea pigs after pretreatment of the application site with SLS. An enhancement of systemic absorption compared with normal skin was different for the four compounds. The concentration in the viable epidermis, however, was not found to differ between intact or SLS-pretreated skin. The most comprehensive summary of published results with the maximization test is detailed in Wahlberg and Boman (1985).

Other Adjuvant Injection Tests

The aim of developing the optimization test (Maurer *et al.*, 1975, 1980; Maurer, 1985) was, to provide a test which was as sensitive as the maximization test, which used standard concentrations for the intradermal injections to permit easy comparison of the sensitizing potential of various compounds, and in which skin reactions could be evaluated objectively.

The experience with this method is based on many different chemical classes (Maurer, 1985, see Table 7.5). The limited use in other laboratories is probably a consequence of the longer duration of the test, because separate intradermal and epidermal challenge applications are regularly performed. The use of two routes of challenge makes it possible to get information about the effects of a substance on intact and diseased skin. This may be particularly

Table 7.6 Comparable data from maximization test and SIAT

	Incidence of positive animals Induction according to selected protocol	
	Maximization (per cent)	SIAT (per cent)
Picryl chloride	100	80
Mercaptobenzothiazole	60	0
Potassium dichromate	100	50
Nickel sulphate	10	10

(Goodwin *et al.*, 1981)

important when testing the active ingredients of dermatics or transdermal therapeutic systems.

In the Freund's Complete Adjuvant test (FCAT), guinea pigs are treated with a total of three adjuvant injections within 9 days of induction and are challenged topically as in the OET protocol (Klecak, 1985). Not much experience has been gained with compounds other than fragrances and comparisons with other tests are difficult also, because the results were published as positive or negative and no threshold is given for a positive result.

A further reduction of the number of adjuvant injections was recommended in the single injection adjuvant test (SIAT) by Goodwin *et al.* (1981) and Goodwin and Johnson (1985). Challenge is performed as in the Buehler test with a single epidermal occlusive application for 6 hours. In the publication of 1985 it is stated that the SIAT is less sensitive than the maximization test of Magnusson and Kligman (see Table 7.6).

Epidermal Tests Combined with FCA Injections

Various methods have been developed which combine topical treatment with the test compound and intradermal injection of adjuvant. The advantages of such a combination are: 1) more human exposure related treatment of the animals, 2) possibility of testing active ingredients alone as well as formulations, 3) attainment of about the same sensitivity of the methods as in the maximization procedure.

Maguire and Chase (1972, Maguire, 1973, 1975) used the combination of adjuvant injections and epidermal application of the test compound in the split adjuvant test. Positive results with benzocaine indicate that the method is sensitive. It is claimed that the method of exposure to the test compound is more "natural" than that used in the maximization test. This is questionable, because the application site has to be shaved before application "till glistening" or pretreated with dry ice. The modified maximization test of Sato (1985) comprises a total of four adjuvant injections on the first treatment day combined with repeated abrasion and occlusive treatments during an induction period of 9 days. The animals are challenged by open topical applications.

The cumulative enhancement test of Tsuchiya *et al.* (1985) includes four epidermal occluded treatments during induction combined with adjuvant injections before the third topical treatment. The challenge is performed open when negative, a second challenge is performed with occlusive treatment.

Maurer and Hess (1989) published a modification of the maximization test. The modification was related only to the first induction procedure in which four adjuvant injections were combined with a 24-hour occlusive treatment. The remainder of the protocol was identical to the standard test of Magnusson and Kligman. The sensititivity of the standard and the modified protocols was comparable, for example:

	Incidence of positive animals	
	Standard Protocol Maximization	Modified Protocol Maximization
Penicillin G	14/19	9–10/10
Benzocaine	1–6/10	4–5/10

Cyclophosphamide is often used to enhance the T cell response in mice. It has not achieved the same value in guinea pigs. One reason may be that cyclophosphamide is less well tolerated in guinea pigs and doses of 250–300 mg/kg result in death (Kashima *et al.* 1993b). The above authors published a short-duration sensitization method that includes the pretreatment of guinea pigs with 200 mg/kg cyclophosphamide 3 days before a combined treatment with adjuvant and occlusive application of the test compound (CA2 test). For the challenge, the animals were treated topically without occlusion (1st and 2nd challenge) or with occlusion (3rd challenge). The sensitivity of the test was comparable with the maximization test. For example:

	Incidence of positive animals			
	CA2 Test Challenge		Maximization Test Challenge	
	1st	2nd	1st	2nd
Citronellal	100%	80%	100%	100%
Benzyl salicylate	100%	80%	20%	30%

Factors Influencing Predictive Value of Guinea Pig Tests

The most complete list of factors that influence the sensitization of guinea pigs was published by Magnusson and Kligman (1970, 1987). Many factors related to guinea pig strain selection and husbandry are not as important as they were

25 years ago, because much standardization has now been achieved. Other factors are still important and some of these are discussed below.

Selection of Vehicles

In most of the cases, two major solvents for intradermal injections are sufficient, saline and the adjuvant itself. As suggested by Magnusson and Kligman (1969), water soluble compounds should be dissolved in saline before the suspension is made with the adjuvant; oil soluble compounds are first dissolved in the adjuvant before being mixed with saline.

For epidermal open applications solvents such as alcohol, mixtures of olive oil and acetone or acetone, ethanol and dimethylacetamide are used. The last mixture, in the proportions of 4:3:3 of dimethylacetamide:acetone:ethanol, has the advantage that applications on the hairy guinea pig skin can be performed easily without running out of the marked area.

Vehicles for epidermal occlusive applications were a subject of much discussion. Yellow or white soft petrolatum is generally recommended by Magnusson and Kligman (1969, 1970). However, it has an acanthotic effect on the epidermis, as do many other vehicles, and skin thickness increase can be observed in guinea pigs after occlusive application without macroscopically visible reactions. Vaseline has been proposed as the optimal vehicle for water as well as oil soluble chemicals. Experiments described by Marzulli and Maibach (1976) and Maurer (1985) showed clearly that there is not a single optimal vehicle for all compounds. However, a clear contact allergen is not positive with one vehicle and negative with another. The vehicle will influence only the incidence of positive animals.

An interesting example is given by Nielsen *et al.* (1992) for nickel sulphate tested in the maximization test. The highest sensitization rate was obtained when lanolin cream was used during induction and water for challenge. The lowest rate was obtained when hydroxypropyl cellulose was used for induction and petrolatum for challenge.

Selection of Induction Concentrations

Magnusson and Kligman (1970) recommended concentrations up to 5 per cent for the intradermal injections and 25 per cent for epidermal treatment if the compound was not a local irritant and was systemically well tolerated.

For the purposes of assessment of occupational risk, the use of one concentration in a larger group of animals has generally been given priority over the use of several doses in smaller groups of animals. If maximal concentrations are used in every step and strong local effects are induced, a diminished response rate may be possible. Schäfer *et al.* (1978) studied the induction of sensitization to para-substituted benzenes using various concentrations. They concluded from the studies with *p*-phenylenediamine that a concentration of 1–2 per cent is the optimal for sensitization and that higher concentrations have an inhibitory effect. A non-linear relationship between concentration and response was also found by Andersen (1987) for formaldehyde in the maximization test. Other examples of dose-dependency are provided by various authors, including Rohold *et al.* (1991a), Li and Aoyama (1992), Liden and Wahlberg (1994), Bronaugh *et al.* (1994) and Nakamura *et al.* (1994).

Roberts and Williams (1982) derived a parameter called relative alkylation index (RAI) based on *in vitro* chemical reactivity, lipophilicity (partition coefficient) and induction dose. They demonstrated with various sultones, that with increasing induction concentration the frequency of reactions could be increased only to a certain level after which the frequency decreases (overload region). Similar results were obtained with alkyl transfer agents (Roberts and Basketter, 1990) tested in the single adjuvant injection test.

The selection of induction concentrations is an important factor. Flexibility should be exercised by authorities when good reasons are given and when the evaluation of major risks are still guaranteed. The selection is dependent also on the aim of the study, such as evaluation of the occupational risk or evaluation of the dose-response relationships for the selection of concentrations in final products. To cover all aspects, the performance of more than one test is recommended.

Reaction Assessment

A repeated area of discussion is the evaluation of reactions. The visual assessment of erythema reactions and the assessment of increases in skinfold thickness by palpation according to grading scales are subjective. However, with a careful selection of challenge concentration, avoiding irritation in controls, chemical depilation of the reaction site in the case of coloured compounds and thorough training of technicians, reproducible results are obtained.

Objective assessments are possible, but they are often time-consuming and do not always distinguish clearly between allergic and irritant reactions. An easy objective way to measure reactions after intradermal injections is the measurement of the reaction diameter and the skinfold thickness with a caliper as it is performed in the optimization test for the induction and challenge reactions (Maurer *et al.*, 1980; Maurer, 1985). To use several parameters instead of skinfold thickness alone has been proposed by Scheper *et al.* (1977) because the influence on the parameters evaluated is compound related. Skinfold thickness measurements after occlusive application of the test compound may cause difficulties because occlusion itself has an acanthotic effect.

Another alternative is histological assessment. This is time consuming and conflicting results have been published on the ability to differentiate between allergic and irritant reactions. Reitamo *et al.* (1981) used naphthyl acetate esterase and endogenous peroxidase as markers for inflammatory cells and could not find a statistical difference between irritant and allergic reactions in patients. Kanerva *et al.* (1983) examined the distribution pattern of Langerhans cells (LC) and their contact with mononuclear cells in sequential biopsies from allergic and irritant reactions. They found no difference in 28 patients tested. Scheynius and Fischer (1986) examined allergic reactions to nickel and cobalt and irritant effects induced by sodium lauryl sulphate in nine patients. The expression of the histocompatibility antigen HLA-DR on keratinocytes was found in nine of 14 allergic reactions but not in irritant ones. The evaluation period was 4 to 20 days after treatment. A difference in the distribution of LC in epidermis and dermis in irritant and allergic reactions was found by Marks *et al.* (1987). In allergic reactions, LC in the dermis were predominantly perivascular 2 to 14 days after treatment; in irritant reactions the LC were widely distributed in the dermis 2 days after treatment but the number of LC was markedly reduced 4 to 7 days afterwards.

Much less work has been done in experimental animals. A useful tool for the differentiation of weak to moderate allergic reactions from irritant reactions in guinea pigs was found by Robinson *et al.* (1990) to be the cutaneous basophil hypersensitivity response. Guinea pigs sensitized with oxazolone, citronellal or cinnamic aldehyde showed a clear quantitative difference in basophil counts compared with animals treated for the first time with the same compounds or with sodium lauryl sulphate. In most cases the values obtained 24 hours after challenge were higher than those measured at 72 hours.

Maurer *et al.* (1991) compared standard histology and immunohistological evaluation of LC in irritant and allergic reactions to DNCB in guinea pigs. With standard histology it was impossible to differentiate between irritant and allergic responses. The immunohistochemical quantification of LC in epidermal sheets or in tissue sections revealed contradictory results and it was concluded that no clear distinction between irritant and allergic reactions could be made.

Various publications have demonstrated differences in the development of irritant and allergic reactions. However, in predictive testing such time-dependent evaluation of the processes is not possible and therefore histology is not an ideal tool in routine sensitization testing.

In recent years non-invasive techniques have been used frequently in man to evaluate objectively skin responses and to differentiate between weak and moderate, or doubtful and weak reactions. As discussed by Li *et al.* (1992) much less experience is available in animals. They used laser doppler flow cytometry in guinea pigs sensitized with DNCB and it was possible to distinguish between a negative and positive response, but not between different intensities of reactions. Evaluation of reactions by a colorimetric method was used by Rohold *et al.* (1991b) in guinea pigs sensitized with nickel sulphate. The variation in responses in negative and weakly positive skin sites made it impossible to differentiate between negative and positive guinea pigs.

A new assessment is to measure the *in vitro* proliferation of lymphocytes from *in vivo* sensitized animals. Kashima *et al.* (1993a) sensitized animals using a short sensitization method (AP2). Lymphocytes and macrophages were cultured *in vitro* and stimulated with ovalbumin and/or haptens. The *in vitro* response of cells from sensitized animals was always greater than the response from untreated control animals. Significant differences were obtained with DNCB, formaldehyde, nickel sulphate, eugenol and cinnamic aldehyde. Good results were obtained with the lymphocyte transformation test (LTT) from animals sensitized with the maximization test. However, Li and Aoyama (1992) presented only data with two haptens, dinitrochlorobenzene and dinitrobenzene sulphonic salt.

Objective assessment of skin reactions has not yet yielded much advantage compared with visual evaluation. Careful selection of challenge concentrations is still an important factor. If doubtful reactions are seen in the majority of reacting animals, it is recommended to repeat the challenge procedure after an additional rest period. During a 1-year period the erythema reactions in 17 out of 100 tested compounds were very weak and the incidence lower than 50 per cent. After a second challenge the results were much clearer; in eight out of 17 compounds the incidence of positive animals increased significantly and in nine of 17 cases the reactivity had clearly diminished (Maurer and Hess, 1989). Every challenge reaction serves also as additional induction treatment. There are, therefore, good scientific reasons to interpret differently results obtained following repeated challenges. The new guidelines include recommendations to repeat challenges when the results are not significantly positive; however, they do not include advice on interpretation of results from different challenges.

Guinea Pig Tests Related to Other Tests

Guinea Pig Versus Mouse

In 1983 the experience with mice was so limited that it was considered that the mouse cannot replace the guinea pig (Maurer, 1983). The introduction of local lymph node assays improved the sensitivity of mouse tests and provided new possibilities for comparison.

In a collaborative study the lymph node responses of guinea pigs and mice were compared (Maurer and Kimber, 1991). The main aim was to determine whether the LLNA was suitable for use in guinea pigs. In general, the response in the mouse was higher and the range of proliferation indices (PI) was larger than in the guinea pig; for some compounds the reverse was the case. Examples of proliferation indices after induction with 2 per cent concentrations and 24-hour *in vitro* incubation were:

	PI in guinea pig	PI in mouse
Oxazolone	6.15	83.4
Cinnamic aldehyde	9.48	3.30
Picryl chloride	2.29	55.8
p-Phenylenediamine	5.27	4.77

Higher responses in guinea pigs were obtained with 48-hour incubations and/or additional stimulation with interleukin-2.

A similar comparative study with metals was published by Ikarashi *et al.* (1992) using guinea pigs, rats and mice. Proliferation indices after sensitization with 2.5 per cent solutions and 24-hour *in vitro* incubations were:

	PI in rat	PI in mice	PI in guinea pig
Potassium dichromate	10.94	4.01	0.97
Cobalt chloride	3.82	3.77	0.75
Nickel sulphate	1.17	2.19	0.77

To achieve optimal responses in different species may require the use of different protocols. This may be the reason why the guinea pig responded less vigorously than the rat or mouse in the studies of Ikarashi *et al.* (1992).

In general, good agreement between guinea pig sensitization tests and the LLNA was found with moderate to strong sensitizers (Ikarashi *et al.*, 1994; Edwards *et al.*, 1994; Basketter and Scholes, 1994). The guinea pig tests were however more sensitive than LLNA with weak sensitizers (see also Chapter 8).

Comparison of Different Guinea Pig Tests

The results for various compounds shown in Tables 7.2–7.5 give an impression of the relative sensitivity of the different methods available. However it is difficult to make clear comparisons when data deriving from different sensitization methods from different laboratories are used. The percentage of positive responses per group with a single chemical tested in various laboratories is quite large. This is particularly the case when weaker allergens are tested (Table 7.7).

The variability of test results between different laboratories is due to the many factors involved in sensitization testing. If protocols are not strictly harmonized between laboratories, such differences must be accepted. What is more important is the reproducibility of the test results over time in the

Table 7.7   Percentage of positive animals per group tested

	Cinnamic aldehyde	Formaldehyde	Penicillin G
Maximization test	60–100%*	18–100%	70–100%
Buehler test	0–50%	30–60%	n.d.
Optimization test	100%	10–100%	33–100%
SIAT	100%	0–70%	80–100%
FCAT	n.d.	20–60%	67–100%
OET	100%	0–50%	0–75%
Draize test	10–20%	10–70%	35%

*Range of positive animals found in various publications, adapted from ECETOC (1990). n.d. = Not determined.

same laboratory and the in-house validation with reference compounds. Only in this way can the sensitizing potential of a new chemical be compared with old data.

Relevance of Guinea Pig Test Data for Man

A positive result in a guinea pig test shows the skin sensitizing potential of the test compound. Magnusson and Kligman (1969) classified compounds according to five classes of potency. Even in the case of a negative result in a guinea pig maximization test, the compound is classified as being a weak sensitizer. The background for this classification is the long experience in occupational dermatology of these two clinicians and the experience that every compound may at some time induce an allergic reaction in man.

In the early phase after introduction of FCA for predictive testing in my laboratory, some of the compounds were additionally tested in repeated insult patch tests (HRIPT) in man. The results obtained showed a good correlation between positive effects after epidermal application in guinea pigs and responses in man (Maurer, 1985). It was apparent also that the number of volunteers is a crucial factor in the HRIPT and that more than 50 volunteers per group should be tested to get an equally good prediction as in guinea pigs.

The correlation between experimental animal and human studies is dependent also on the protocol used. A much better correlation between FCA tests and predictive human tests was observed by Marzulli and Maguire (Table 7.8). The difference in intensity of adjuvant and non-adjuvant tests has been taken into account for the labelling of compounds according to EEC Commission Directive (EEC, 1993). Any compound inducing at least 30 per cent positive animals in an adjuvant test must be labelled with the risk phrase

Table 7.8 Correlation between predictive animal and predictive human tests

Guinea pig protocol	Assessment with predictive human tests		
	Agreement	False positive	False negative
Draize	14	1	15
Buehler	10	0	20
Maximization	29	0	1
Split adjuvant test	22	2	6

Adapted from Marzulli and Maguire (1987).

Table 7.9A Correlation between predictive animal tests and clinical experience

Animal test	Clinical experience			
	No clinical cases	Listed in epidemiological studies	Listed for special groups	Single cases
Positive adjuvant tests (319)	62	89	133	145
Negative adjuvant tests (68)	10	22	33	26
Positive non-adjuvant tests (152)	19	39	70	86
Negative non-adjuvant tests (111)	9	43	55	46

Results of the assessment of all compounds listed in table of Klaschka and Vossmann (1994).

Table 7.9B

Animal test	Clinical experience		
	Listed in epidemiological studies	Listed for special groups	Single cases
Positive adjuvant tests (54)	24	29	36
Negative adjuvant tests (4)	2	1	4
Positive non-adjuvant tests (45)	17	29	31
Negative non-adjuvant tests (13)	10	5	12

Results of the assessment of 110 compounds classified as the most relevant allergens by the working group.

R43. In the case of a non-adjuvant test 15 per cent positives are sufficient.

Some years ago, a working group of the health authorities in Berlin started the evaluation of contact allergens from the published literature. Data for nearly a thousand compounds was summarized in a tabulated form which included data from predictive animal studies, predictive human studies and clinical experience data. The full list was published in 1994 (Klaschka and Vossmann, 1994). Table 7.9 summarizes a first assessment of animal and clinical data. The significance of the animal data to be included in the table as positive or negative was judged by the authors and not according to the EEC classification criteria. The clinical data were categorized in three ways, as data from epidemiological evaluation, as descriptions of single cases and as data from specific collectives. Simultaneous citations in the clinical categories were possible for a single compound and therefore the total number of clinical citations is not identical to the total number of animal tests. Test results of 387 adjuvant tests and 263 non-adjuvant tests are included in the table of Klaschka and Vossmann. 319 adjuvant tests were positive and 68 were negative. For 62 chemicals out of the 319 positive adjuvant tests, no clinical data is as yet published. It is not known how many of the 62 compounds ever came to the market. On the other hand, clinical results were published for the majority of compounds out of 111 chemicals with negative non-adjuvant tests results. The general impression was that adjuvant tests overestimate the risk for sensitization and that non-adjuvant tests underestimate the risk for man. In the meantime, the compounds listed in the tables of Klaschka and Vossmann (1994) were classified by the working group in four categories according to their clinical significance. The list of the most relevant compounds and a short report for each compound will be published soon by the German authorities (Bundesamt für gesundheitlichen Verbraucherschutz und Veterinärwesen.). For the 110 most relevant compounds, 54 of 58 published results of adjuvant tests were positive, four compounds were false negative in animal tests. The results of non-adjuvant tests were 45 positive out of 58 tested (Table 7.10). This second list showed a much better correlation between animal tests and clinical experience. Additionally, it confirmed that predictive non-adjuvant tests underestimate the risk for sensitization in man.

References

ANDERSEN, K.E., 1987, Testing for contact allergy in experimental animals, *Pharmacol. & Toxicol.* **61**, 1–8.

ANDERSEN, K.E., MAIBACH, H.I., 1985, Contact allergy, predictive tests in guinea pigs, Karger, Basel.

BASKETTER, D.A., SCHOLES, E.W., 1992, Comparison of the local lymph node assay with the guinea pig maximization test for the detection of a range of contact allergens, *Food Chem. Toxicol.*, **30**, 65–9.

BASKETTER, D.A., SELBIE, E., SCHOLES, E.W., Lees, D., KIMBER, I., BOTHAM,

P.A., 1993, Results with OECD recommended positive control sensitizers in the maximization, Buehler and local lymph node assays, *Food Chem. Toxicol.* **31**, 63–7.

BRONAUGH, R.L., ROBERTS, C.D., McCOY, J.L., 1994, Dose-response relationship in skin sensitization, *Food. Chem. Toxic.*, **32**, 113–7.

BUEHLER, E. V., 1965, Delayed contact hypersensitivity in the guinea pig, *Arch. Dermatol.*, **91**, 171–7.

1994, Occlusive patch method for skin sensitization in guinea pigs: the Buehler method, *Food Chem. Toxic.*, **32**, 97–101.

BUEHLER, E.V., GRIFFITH, J.F., 1975, Experimental skin sensitization in the guinea pig and man, in: Animal Models in Dermatology, H.I. Maibach (ed.), Churchill Livingstone, Edinburgh, pp. 56–66.

DRAIZE, J.H., 1959, Intracutaneous sensitisation test on guinea pigs, in Association of Food and Drug Officials of the United States, Austin, Texas, Appraisal of the safety of chemicals in food and cosmetics.

DRAIZE, J.H., WOODWARD, G., CALVERY, H.O., 1944, Methods for the study of irritation and toxicity of substances applied topically to the skin and mucous membranes, *J. Pharms. Exp. Therap.*, **82**, 377–89.

ECETOC, 1990, European Chemical Industry Ecology & Toxicology Centre, Monograph No. 14, Skin Sensitization.

EDWARDS, D.A., SORANNO, T.M., AMORUSO, M.A., HOUSE, R.V., TUMMEY, A.C., TRIMMER, G.W., THOMAS, P.T., RIBEIRO, P.L., 1994, Screening petrochemicals for contact hypersensitivity potential: a comparison of the murine local lymph node assay with guinea pig and human test data, *Fund. Appl. Toxicol.*, **23**, 179–87.

EEC, 1984, Commission Directive of 25 April 1984 adapting to technical progress for the sixth time Council Directive 67/548/EEC on the laws, regulations and administrative provisions relating to the classification, packaging and labelling of dangerous substances, *Off. J. Europ. Commun.*, L 251, Vol. **27**, 113.

1992, Commission Directive of 29 December 1992 adapting to technical progress for the 17th time Council Directive on laws, regulations and administrative provisions relating to classification, packaging and labelling of dangerous substances, *Off. J. Europ. Commun.*, L 383 A, 131–6.

1993, Annexes I, II, III and IV to Commission Directive 93/21/EEC of 27 April 1993 adapting to technical progress for the 18th time Council Directive 67/548/EEC on the approximation of the laws, regulations and administrative provisions relating to the classification, packaging and labelling of dangerous substances, *Off. J. Europ. Commun.*, L 110 A, **36**, 1–86.

GOODWIN, B.F.J., CREWEL, R.W.R., JOHNSON, A.W., 1981, A comparison of three guinea-pig sensitization procedures for the detection of 19 reported human contact sensitizers, *Contact Dermatitis*, **7**, 248–58.

GOODWIN, B.F.J., JOHNSON, A.W., 1985, Single injection adjuvant test, *Curr. Probl. Derm.*, **14**, 201–7.

IKARASHI, Y., OHNO, K., TSUCHIYA, T., NAKAMURA. A., 1992, Differences of draining lymph node cell proliferation among mice, rats and guinea pigs following exposure to metal allergens, *Toxicology*, **76**, 283–92.

1994, Assessment of contact sensitivity of four thiourea rubber accelerators: comparison of two mouse lymph node assays with the guinea pig maximization test, *Food Chem. Toxicol.* **32**, 1067–72.

JOHNSON, A.W., GOODWIN, B.F.J., 1985, The Draize test and modifications, *Curr. Probl. Derm.*, **14**, 31–8.

KANERVA, L., RANKI, A., MUSTAKALLIO, K., LAUHARANTA, J., 1983, Langerhans cell-mononuclear cell contacts are not specific for allergy in patch tests, *Brit. J. Dermatol.*, **109**, Suppl. 25, 64–7.

KASHIMA, R., OKADA, J., IKEDA, Y., YOSHIZUKA, N., 1993a, Challenge assay in vitro using lymphocyte blastogenesis for the contact hypersensitivity assay, *Food Chem. Toxicol.*, **31**, 759–66.

KASHIMA, R., OYAKE, Y., OKADA, J., IKEDA, Y., 1993b, Studies of new short-period method for delayed contact hypersensitivity assay in the guinea pig, studies of the enhancement effect of cyclophosphamide, *Contact Dermatitis*, **29**, 26–32.

KLASCHKA, F., VOSSMANN, D., 1994, Kontaktallergene, Chemisch, klinische und experimentelle Daten (Allergen-Liste), ESV, Berlin.

KLECAK, G., 1985, The Freund's complete adjuvant test and the open epicutaneous test, *Curr. Probl. Derm.*, **14**, 152–71.

KLECAK. G., GELEICK, H., FREY, J. R., 1977, Screening of fragrance materials for allergenicity in the guinea pig, Comparison of four testing methods, *J. Soc. Cosmet. Chem.*, **28**, 53–64.

KNUDSEN, B.B., WAHLBERG, J.E., ANDERSEN, I., MENNE, T., 1993, Classification of contact allergens, *Dermatosen*, **41**, 5–9.

LI, Q., AOYAMA, K., 1992, Study of dose-response relationship in contact sensitivity using an in vitro assay, *Contact Dermatitis*, **27**, 16–21.

LI, Q., AOYAMA, K., MATSUSHITA, T., 1992, Evaluation of contact allergy to chemicals using laser Doppler flowmetry (LDF) technique, *Contact Dermatitis*, **26**, 27–33.

LIDEN, C., WAHLBERG, J.E., 1994, Cross-reactivity to metal compounds studied in guinea pig induced with chromate or cobalt, *Acta Derm. Venereol.*, **74**, 341–3.

MAGNUSSON, B., KLIGMAN, A.M., 1969, The identification of contact allergens by animal assay. The guinea pig maximization test, *J. Invest. Dermatol.*, **52**, 268–76.

MAGNUSSON, B., KLIGMAN, A.M., 1970, Allergic Contact Dermatitis in the Guinea Pig, Charles C. Thomas, Springfield.

MAGNUSSON, B., KLIGMAN, A. M., 1987, Factors influencing allergic contact sensitization, in: Dermatotoxicology 3rd edition, F.N. Marzulli, H.I. Maibach, (eds.), Hemisphere Publ. Co., Cambridge.

MAGUIRE, H.C., 1973, The bioassay of contact allergens in the guinea pig, *J. Soc. Cosmet. Chem.*, **24**, 151–62.

MAGUIRE H.C., 1975, Estimation of the allergenicity of prospective human contact sensitizers in the guinea pig, in: Animal Models in Dermatology, H.I. Maibach, (ed.), Churchill Livingstone, Edinburgh, pp. 67–75.

MAGUIRE, H.C., CHASE, M.W., 1972, Studies on the sensitization of animals with simple chemical compounds, *J. Exp. Med.*, **135**, 357–75.

MARKS, J.G., ZAINO, R.J., BRESSLER, M. F., WILLIAMS, J.V., 1987, Changes in lymphocyte and Langerhans cell populations in allergic and irritant contact dermatitis, *Int. J. Dermatol.*, **26**, 354–7.

MARZULLI, F.N., MAIBACH, H.I., 1976, Effects of vehicles and elicitation concentration in contact dermatitis testing, *Contact Dermatitis*, **2**, 325–9.

1987, Dermatotoxicology, 3rd edition, Hemisphere Publ. Corp., Washington.

MARZULLI, F., MAGUIRE, H.C., 1987, Validation of guinea pig tests for skin hypersensitivity, in: Dermatotoxicology, 3rd edition, F.N. Marzulli, H.I. Maibach (eds.), Hemisphere Publ. Co., Washington pp. 277–90.

MAURER, T., 1983, Contact and Photocontact Allergens, A Manual of Predictive Test Methods, Marcel Dekker Inc., New York.

1985, The optimization test, *Curr. Probl. Derm.*, **14**, 114–51.

MAURER, T., KIMBER, I., 1991, Draining lymph node cell activation in guinea pigs: comparisons with the murine local lymph node assay, *Toxicol.*, **69**, 209–18.

MAURER, T., THOMANN, P., WEIRICH, E.G., HESS, R., 1975, The optimization test in the guinea pig, *Agents and Actions*, **5**, 174–9.

MAURER, T., WEIRICH, E.G., HESS, R., 1980, The optimization test in the guinea pig in relation to other predictive sensitization methods, *Toxicol.*, **15**, 163–71.

MAURER, T., HESS, R., 1989, The maximization test for skin sensitization potential – updating the standard protocol and validation of a modified protocol, *Food. Chem. Toxicol*, **27**, 807–11.

MAURER, T., GERMER, M., KRINKE, A., 1991, Does the immunohistochemical detection of Langerhans cell help in the differential diagnosis of irritative and allergic skin reactions?, *Progress in Histo- and Cytochem.*, **23**, 256–62.

NAKAMURA, A., MOMMA, J., SEKIGUCHI, H., NODA, I., YAMANO, T., KANIWA, M.-A., KOJIMA, S., TSUDA, M., KUROKAWA, Y., 1994, A new protocol and criteria for quantitative determination of sensitization potencies of chemicals by guinea pig maximization test, *Contact Dermatitis*, **31**, 72–85.

NIELSEN, G.D., ROHOLD, A.E., ANDERSEN, K.E., 1992, Nickel contact sensitivity in the guinea pig, an efficient open application method, *Acta Derm. Venereol.*, **72**, 45–8.

OECD (Organization for Economic Cooperation and Development), 1981, OECD Guideline for Testing of Chemicals, No. 406, Skin Sensitization.

1992, OECD Guideline for Testing of Chemicals, adopted by the Council on July 17, Skin Sensitization.

POLIKANDRITOU, M., CONINE D., 1985, Enhancement of the sensitivity of the Buehler method by use of the Hill Top Chamber®, *J. Soc. Cosmet. Chem.*, **36**, 159–68.

REITAMO, S., TOVANEN, E., KONTTINEN, Y.T., KÄYHKÖ, K., FÖRSTRÖM, L., SALO, O.P., 1981, Allergic and toxic contact dermatitis: inflammatory cell subtypes in epicutaneous test reactions, *Brit. J. Dermatol.*, **105**, 521–7.

ROBERTS, D.W., BASKETTER, D.A., 1990, A quantitative structure activity/dose response relationship for contact allergic potential of alkyl group transfer agents, *Contact Dermatitis*, **23**, 331–5.

ROBERTS, D.W., WILLIAMS, D.L., 1982, The derivation of quantitative correlations between skin sensitisation and physico-chemical parameters for alkylating agents, and their application to experimental data for sultones, *J. Theor. Biol.*, **99**, 807–25.

ROBINSON, M.K., NUSAIR, T. L., FLETCHER, E.R., RITZ, H. L., 1990, A review of the Buehler guinea pig skin sensitization test and its use in a risk assessment process for human skin sensitization, *Toxicol.*, **61**, 91–107.

ROBINSON, M.K., FLETCHER, E. R., JOHNSON, G.R., WYDER, W.E., MAURER, J.K., 1990, Value of the cutaneous basophil hypersensitivity (CBH) response for distinguishing weak contact sensitization from irritation reactions in the guinea pig, *J. Invest. Dermatol.*, **94**, 636–43.

ROHOLD, A.E., NIELSEN, G. D., ANDERSEN, K. E., 1991a, Nickel-sulphate-induced contact dermatitis in the guinea pig maximization test: a dose-response study, *Contact Dermatitis*, **24**, 35–9.

1991b, Colorimetric quantification of erythema in the guinea pig maximization test, *Contact Dermatitis*, **24**, 373–4.

SATO, Y., Modified guinea pig maximization test, *Curr. Probl. Derm.*, **14**, 193–200.

SCHÄFER, U., METZ, J., PEVNY, I., RÖCKL, H., 1978, Sensibilisierungsversuche an Meerschweinchen mit fünf parasubstituierten Benzolderivaten, *Arch. Derm. Res.*, **261**, 153–61.

SCHEPER, R.J., NOBLE, B., PARKER, D., TURK, J.L., 1977, The value of an assessment of erythema and increase in thickness of the skin reaction for a full appreciation of the nature of delayed hypersensitivity in the guinea pig, *Int. Arch. Allergy Appl. Immunol.*, **54**, 58–66.

SCHEYNIUS, A., FISCHER, T., 1986, Phenotypic difference between allergic and irritant patch test reactions in man, *Contact Dermatitis*, **14**, 297–302.

SCHLEDE, E., MAURER, T., POTOKAR, M., SCHMIDT, W.M., SCHULZ, K.H., ROLL, R., KAYSER, D., 1989, A differentiated approach to testing skin sensitization, *Arch. Toxicol.*, **63**, 81–4.

SHARP, D.W., 1978, The sensitization potential of some perfume ingredients tested using a modified Draize procedure, *Toxicol.*, **9**, 261–71.

STEVENS, M.A., 1967, Use of the albino guinea pig to detect the skin sensitizing ability of chemicals, *Brit. J. Ind. Med.*, **24**, 189–202.

TSUCHIYA, S., KONDO, M., OKAMOTO, K., TAKASE, Y., 1985, The cumulative contact enhancement test, *Curr. Probl. Derm.*, **14**, 208–19.

VOSS, J.G., 1958, Skin sensitization by mercaptans of low molecular weight, *J. Invest. Dermatol.*, **31**, 273–9.

WAHLBERG, J.E., BOMAN, A., 1985, Guinea pig maximization test, *Curr. Probl. Derm.*, **14**, 59–106.

WEIRICH, E.G., 1962, Zur Methodik der tierexperimentellen Prüfung kosmet. Dermatika auf ihre Haurverträglichkeit. Deutsche Gesellschaft für Fettwissenschaften, Düsseldorf.

WILHELM, K.P., SURBER, CH., MAIBACH, H.I., 1991, Effect of sodium lauryl sulphate-induced skin irritation on in vivo percutaneous penetration of four drugs, *J. Invest. Dermatol.*, **97**, 927–32.

8

Mouse Predictive Tests

I. KIMBER

Zeneca Central Toxicology Laboratory, Macclesfield

Introduction

As described in the previous chapter, it is the guinea pig that has traditionally represented the species of choice for the prospective assessment of contact sensitizing potential. There has in recent years, however, been a growing interest in the mouse for experimental studies of contact sensitization and, latterly, for the identification of contact allergens. The popularity of the mouse dates from the development of quantitative methods for the measurement of contact hypersensitivity reactions in this species. The first and still most popular of these methods was the measurement of challenge-induced increases in the ear thickness of previously sensitized mice, described originally by Asherson and Ptak in 1968. While other methods have been developed and used, notably the incorporation of radiolabelled cells or proteins into the challenge site (Sabbadini *et al.*, 1974; Eipert and Miller, 1975; Mekori *et al.*, 1986), it was the convenience of ear thickness measurements that facilitated the more extensive use of mice in investigative studies. Such studies have borne fruit and have contributed significantly to our understanding of the immunobiological processes that characterize contact sensitization. It is not surprising, therefore, that in recent years there has been an increasing interest in the use of mice for the toxicological assessment of skin sensitizing potential. It is the purpose of this chapter to describe the methods available and the progress that has been made.

Mouse Ear Swelling Test

The first structured approach to evaluation of skin sensitizing activity as a function of challenge-induced increases in ear thickness resulted in the description of the mouse ear swelling test or MEST (Gad *et al.*, 1986). In its original form the MEST incorporated a rigorous induction regime comprising the repeated application (daily for four consecutive days) of test material to tape-stripped abdominal skin, the treatment site having been prepared previously by the intradermal administration of Freund's Complete Adjuvant to enhance immunogenicity. Control mice were treated in an identical manner with vehicle alone. Seven days following completion of the induction procedure both test and control animals were treated on the dorsum of one ear with the test material and on the contralateral ear with vehicle. Concentrations of the test agent used for challenge were selected on the basis of prior sighting studies for lack of irritant activity. Induced changes in ear thickness were measured 1 and 2 days after challenge (Gad *et al.*, 1986). This method was used to evaluate more than 70 chemicals which, on the basis of guinea pig and/or human studies, were known to display varying skin sensitizing potential. The results of this first validation study were encouraging, although with some sensitizing chemicals only modest changes in ear thickness were recorded (Gad *et al.*, 1986). A similar method, also incorporating treatment with adjuvant, the mouse ear sensitization assay, was described by Descotes in 1988. In two subsequent investigations doubts were raised about the sensitivity of the MEST and its ability to identify chemicals with weak to moderate skin sensitizing activity (Cornacoff *et al.*, 1988; Dunn *et al.*, 1990). However, in at least one of these studies a modification of the original procedure was used (Cornacoff *et al.*, 1988).

It has been known for some time that increased dietary vitamin A will augment cell-mediated immune responses and contact hypersensitivity (Malkovsky 1983a, b; Miller *et al.*, 1984) and it has been proposed that the maintenance of mice on diets supplemented with vitamin A acetate may increase the sensitivity of MEST-like methods (Maisey and Miller, 1986). Employing this phenomenon, Thorne and colleagues described a 'non-invasive' mouse ear swelling assay (MESA) in which vitamin A-enriched diets were used in place of intradermal injections of adjuvant and tape stripping as a means of ensuring sufficient sensitivity (Thorne *et al.*, 1991a, b). The findings of Thorne *et al.* were endorsed subsequently by an independent study in which it was observed that the MEST was able to detect what were considered to be three comparatively weak chemical sensitizers (glutaraldehyde, formaldehyde and an azo dye) only if mice were fed on diet supplemented with vitamin A (Sailstad *et al.*, 1993). In a recent modification of the original MEST protocol Gad (1994) has proposed the use of vitamin A as a dietary supplement together with adjuvant injection during the induction stage. This modified design for the MEST procedure is illustrated in Figure 8.1. The question raised is whether an aggressive induction protocol is necessary to provide the degree of sensitivity required to identify the majority of skin sensitizing chemicals. Variations of the MEST have been tabulated recently by Garrigue *et al.* (1994) who themselves favour an induction regime comprising only topical application of the test material to

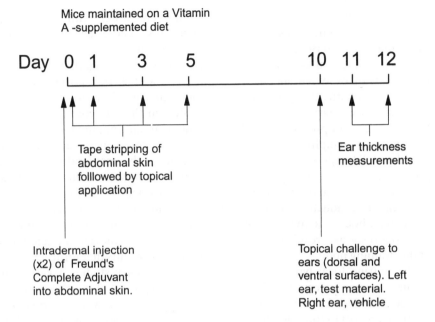

Figure 8.1 Design of a revised mouse ear swelling test (MEST) (modified from Gad, 1994)

shaved backs of mice on three consecutive days without the use of vitamin A-enriched diets. Despite some uncertainty about the need for adjuvant and the advantages resulting from the use of dietary vitamin A and epidermal tape stripping, the basic approach of MEST-type methods is sound. There is a need, however, to ensure that in any variant of this method there is sufficient sensitivity to identify accurately a range of chemical allergens, including those that are considered to exhibit only comparatively weak skin sensitizing potential. A constraint presently in assessing the relative utility of different MEST procedures is that in many of the investigations cited above only a very small number of chemicals has been tested and frequently the materials selected have significant sensitizing activity.

The Local Lymph Node Assay

In common with guinea pig predictive tests, the MEST and related assays are based upon the evaluation of challenge-induced dermal reactions in previously sensitized animals. A method that seeks instead to identify chemical allergens as a function of events that characterize the induction phase of skin sensitization is the local lymph node assay. There is now available detailed information about the cellular and molecular processes that result in contact sensitization following first encounter with a chemical allergen on the skin. These events have been reviewed elsewhere (Kimber, 1992) and are described in Chapter 2 of this volume.

Chemical allergen associates with resident epidermal Langerhans cells, and possibly with other cutaneous dendritic cells, and is transported, via the afferent lymphatics, to lymph nodes draining the site of exposure. Dendritic cells that have migrated from the skin localize in the paracortical region of lymph nodes and present the inducing hapten, in an immunogenic form, to responsive T lymphocytes, that as a result become activated. Antigen-stimulated T lymphocytes divide and differentiate; the proliferative response providing an expanded population of allergen-responsive cells that will initiate contact hypersensitivity reactions following subsequent exposure to the same chemical. The induction phase of skin sensitization is therefore characterized by T lymphocyte activation and proliferation in draining lymph nodes. Vigorous responses result also in a substantial increase in the size and cellularity of the draining node. It is the measurement of these events that forms the basis of the murine local lymph node assay. In preliminary studies a variety of parameters was measured following the topical exposure of mice to chemical allergens. Induced changes in draining lymph node weight were recorded and the frequency of pyroninophilic (activated) lymph node cells was measured. In addition the proliferative activity of lymph node cells was measured *in vitro* following culture with radiolabelled thymidine. Proliferative responses were evaluated in the presence or absence of a source of interleukin 2 (IL-2), a T cell growth factor that stimulates and maintains cell division by activated T lymphocytes (Kimber *et al.*, 1986; Oliver *et al.*, 1986; Kimber and Weisenberger, 1989a). It was found that potent chemical allergens caused changes in all parameters measured, inducing increased lymph node weight, the appearance of pyroninophilic cells and vigorous lymph node cell proliferative responses that were augmented in the presence of IL-2. With weaker allergens, however, changes in node weight were modest or virtually undetectable and it was concluded that lymph node cell proliferative responses represented the most robust and sensitive correlate of skin sensitizing activity (Kimber and Weisenberger, 1989a). For this reason subsequent studies focused upon measurement of hyperplastic responses induced in draining nodes. The available evidence supports the selection of lymph node cell proliferation as a relevant marker of skin sensitization. It has been found that the vigour of lymph node cell proliferative responses correlates closely in mice with the extent to which sensitization will develop (Kimber and Dearman, 1991) and that impaired T lymphocyte proliferation during the induction stage will inhibit sensitization and the elicitation of dermal hypersensitivity reactions following challenge (Kimber *et al.*, 1989b).

With the purpose of obviating the need for tissue culture a modified local lymph node assay was developed in which proliferative activity is measured *in situ* following the intravenous injection of treated mice with radiolabelled thymidine (Kimber *et al.*, 1989a; Kimber and Weisenberger, 1989b). It is this assay, in a slightly modified form, that has been the subject of extensive comparisons with guinea pig predictive tests, the MEST and the results of human maximization tests (Kimber *et al.*, 1990b, 1991b, 1994; Basketter and Scholes, 1992, Basketter *et al.*, 1991, 1992, 1993, 1994). Taken together these analyses have shown the local lymph node assay to be a reliable method for the identification of significant skin sensitizing chemicals, although it has frequently proven difficult, but not impossible (Gerberick *et al.*, 1992), to elicit positive responses with nickel salts. With respect to nickel the MEST also has yielded variable results (Gad *et al.*, 1986; Cornacoff *et al.*, 1988; Dunn *et al.*, 1990). The local lymph node assay has been evaluated also within the context of national and international interlaboratory trials. The results of these have shown the method to be robust and to generate comparable results in the independent laboratories (Kimber *et al.*, 1991b, 1995; Basketter *et al.*, 1991; Scholes *et al.*, 1992; Kimber and Basketter, 1992). The development, validation and application of the local lymph node assay have been reviewed in detail elsewhere (Kimber, 1989, 1993; Kimber and Basketter, 1992; Kimber and Dearman 1993, 1994; Kimber *et al.*, 1994). In summary the assay offers a number of advantages compared with guinea pig test methods, not least of which are that local lymph node assay is relatively rapid and cost-effective to perform. In addition, the read-out is objective and quantitative and, unlike some of the more sensitive guinea pig methods and the original MEST, does not require the use of adjuvant. Exposure of mice is via the relevant route and the assay can be used for the evaluation of coloured materials and dyestuffs which may cause interpretative difficulties in guinea pig assays where activity is measured usually as a function of challenge-induced erythematous reactions.

Presently the assay is performed as follows. Groups of CBA/Ca strain mice are exposed daily, for three consecutive days, to various concentrations of the test material or to an equivalent volume of the relevant vehicle alone. Chemicals are applied to the dorsum of both ears. Five days following the initiation of exposure mice are injected intravenously with radiolabelled (^{3}H) thymidine. Animals are sacrificed 5 hours later and the draining auricular lymph nodes isolated and pooled for each experimental group. Single cell suspensions of lymph node cells are prepared by mechanical disaggregation and processed for liquid scintillation counting. The method is shown diagrammatically in Figure 8.2. Chemicals are classified either as 'sensitizers' or 'not strong sensitizers' according to the level of thymidine incorporation. Currently, the criterion for a positive response, and classification as 'sensitizer', is that one or more concentrations of the test material should elicit a three-fold or greater increase in isotope incorporation compared with concurrent vehicle controls. The decision to select a stimulation index of 3 as an arbitrary indicator of sensitizing activity was made on the basis of investigations performed with a wide range of chemicals. Although there is no reason to suppose that this degree of immune stimulation in draining lymph nodes necessarily represents a threshold for the induction of skin

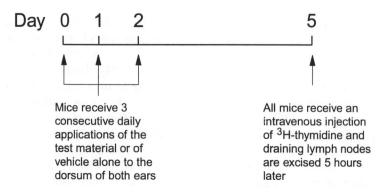

Figure 8.2 Design of the local lymph node assay (from Kimber and Basketter, 1992; Kimber *et al.*, 1994)

sensitization, the use of an index of 3 has proven valuable and accurate in the majority of instances.

In initial studies of the local lymph node assay, and employing a stimulation index of 3 as being indicative of allergenic potential, it was found that skin irritants considered not to cause contact sensitization failed to elicit positive responses in the local lymph node assay. With increasing experience using a wider range of test materials, and following minor changes in assay design, it has become apparent that some, but by no means all, skin irritants induce relatively low levels of proliferative activity in draining nodes that can result in a stimulation index of 3 or greater. Thus, for instance, some investigators have found sodium lauryl sulphate to provoke positive responses in the local lymph node assay (Basketter *et al.*, 1994; Montelius *et al.*, 1994), while others using a standard or modified protocol, have not (Pfennig and Ziegler, 1991; Rodenberger *et al.*, 1993; Ikarashi *et al.*, 1993c). The weight of evidence indicates that some irritant chemicals do indeed display a usually limited potential to provoke local lymph node responses. While the reasons for this are currently unclear it is possible that some skin irritants are able to induce in the epidermis the changes required for the migration of Langerhans cells to draining lymph nodes. If these Langerhans cells serve to transport environmental antigens from the skin to the nodes then some immuno-stimulatory activity might be expected (Cumberbatch *et al.*, 1993). Alternatively, it might be the case that in some instances chemicals considered to act only as cutaneous irritants may in reality have some limited potential to induce skin sensitization (Stringer *et al.*, 1991). This issue clearly warrants further investigation. At present, however, the 'noise' created by some skin irritants appears not to pose any significant interpretative difficulties.

Recently the standard local lymph node assay, or modifications of the test, have been used to evaluate the skin sensitizing activity of discrete chemical classes including biocides, rubber additives and accelerators, petrochemicals, dyes, metal salts and chemical mutagens (Botham *et al.*, 1991; Ikarashi *et al.*, 1992, 1993a, c; 1994; Ashby *et al.*, 1993; Edwards *et al.*, 1994; Sailstad *et al.*, 1994; Potter and Hazelton, 1995).

Attempts have been made to increase the sensitivity of the local lymph node assay. These range from comparatively modest changes in assay design, such as the incorporation of pretreatment on the flank prior to ear exposure, an increase in the number of applications to the ears or homogenization of whole lymph nodes (Kimber and Weisenberger, 1991; Gerberick *et al.*, 1992; Potter and Hazelton, 1995) to the use of an aggressive exposure regime comprising intradermal injection of the test material with Freund's Complete Adjuvant (Ikarashi *et al.*, 1993b, 1994). While, in the latter case, the investigators claimed increased sensitivity, it must be borne in mind that intradermal administration and the requirement for adjuvant negates some of the advantages (simplicity and the relevance of the route of exposure) that the standard method offers. An interesting recent development has been the suggestion that diets enriched in vitamin A acetate may increase the vigour of lymph node cell proliferative responses induced in mice by sensitizing chemicals. It was found that in some instances maintenance of mice for 3 weeks on a diet supplemented with vitamin A acetate permitted the induction of positive local lymph node assay responses at concentrations of chemical allergens which failed to register positive when mice fed on standard diets were used (Sailstad *et al.*, 1995).

Clearly, there is some interest in the development of alternative procedures for the conduct of the local lymph node assay and it will be of importance to determine whether any of the modifications proposed, either singly or in combination, offer tangible advantages with respect to sensitivity or selectivity. All the variants of the standard local lymph node assay described above have in common the measurement of induced lymph node cell proliferative responses (either *in situ* or following culture) as the end-point of the test. It may be possible now, however, to consider as correlates of lymph node activation biological responses other than proliferative activity. Particularly attractive in this respect is the development of a molecular read-out for the assay based upon the stimulation by chemical allergens of cytokine production by draining lymph node cells. Immune activation is associated with the rapid stimulation of cytokine production and it has been shown that chemical allergens will induce the synthesis and secretion by draining lymph node cells of a variety of cytokines including interleukins 1β, 2, 3, 4 and 6 (IL-1β, IL-2, IL-3, IL-4 and IL-6), granulocyte/macrophage colony-stimulating factor (GM-CSF) and interferon-γ (IFN-γ) (Marcinkiewicz and Chain, 1989, 1990; Hopkins *et al.*, 1990; Kimber *et al.*, 1992; Hope *et al.*, 1994). Investigations have been conducted recently to determine whether one such product of allergen-activated lymph node cells, the multifunctional cytokine IL-6, provides a sensitive and reliable correlate of skin sensitizing potential (Dearman *et al.*, 1993, 1994; Dearman and Kimber, 1994; Hilton *et al.*, 1994). The results of those studies, in which IL-6 was measured by enzyme-linked immunosorbent assay in the supernants of cultured lymph node cells, demonstrated that while the method was robust, yielding equivalent results in two independent laboratories (Dearman *et al.*, 1994), the secretion of detectable concentrations of this cytokine was an insufficiently sensitive marker of sensitizing activity for routine use in place of the standard procedure. The exercise did, however, serve to emphasize the potential advantages associated with the evaluation of molecular, rather than cellular, correlates of lymph node activation. Thus, for instance batch analyses can be performed permitting direct comparisons between experiments. In addition, repeat analyses can be conducted in the same and/or independent laboratories. Although IL-6 measurements, at least as conducted in the investigations cited above, may not provide sufficient sensitivity for the identification of a wide range of contact allergens, this may not be the case for other cytokine products of lymph node cells (or indeed for IL-6 itself should more sensitive analytical techniques be employed). Of special interest may be IFN-γ, a product of activated T lymphocytes. This cytokine is synthesized by a functional subpopulation of $CD4^+$ T helper (Th) cells, designated Th1, and it is Th1 cells that are primarily responsible for the development and expression of contact sensitization. There is undoubtedly still some way to go in determining whether the synthesis of cytokines or other products of activated lymph node cells can replace the measurement of proliferative responses in the local lymph node assay. Nevertheless it is an area worthy of further investigation.

Systemic Evaluation of Contact Hypersensitivity

Contact hypersensitivity may be defined as a local dermal inflammatory reaction which can be elicited in susceptible (sensitized) individuals at concentrations of the inducing chemical allergen that fail to provoke similar lesions in non-sensitized controls. Although the inflammatory response induced is local and restricted to the site of challenge, it may be assumed that there will be some systemic serological manifestations of the reaction. There have been some attempts to develop in mice serological methods for the evaluation of contact hypersensitivity reactions. Inflammatory responses are associated with changes in the serum concentration of acute phase proteins. It has been demonstrated that the elicitation of contact reactions in mice sensitized previously with chemicals such as oxazolone and picryl chloride is associated with significant increases in the serum concentration of two acute phase proteins, haptoglobin and serum amyloid A. Similar changes were not observed following challenge, under identical conditions, of non-sensitized mice (Kimber *et al.*, 1989c). Increases in the hepatic synthesis and plasma concentration of acute phase proteins are regulated by cytokines and, in particular, by IL-6. Consistent with this is the fact that sensitization and challenge of mice with oxazolone was found to result also in a time-dependent increase in the concentration of plasma IL-6 (Kimber *et al.*, 1990a). Similarly, the elicitation of contact reactions in mice is associated with a significant elevation of serum histamine concentrations (Kimber *et al.*, 1991a). While such systemic manifestations of local contact hypersensitivity reactions are of some value in the measurement of responses to strong sensitizing chemicals, induced changes in the serum concentration of IL-6, acute phase proteins and histamine are insufficiently vigorous for use in standard screening methods.

Conclusions

In the last 10 years much attention has focused on the development in the mouse of predictive methods for the assessment of skin sensitizing activity. Some considerable progress has been made and currently two tests, the MEST and the local lymph node assay, have been recognized by the Organization for Economic Cooperation and Development (OECD) as being suitable for screening chemicals as the first stage in an assessment process (OECD, 1992). It is anticipated that a continuing willingness to apply to exploratory toxicology our increasing understanding of the immunobiological responses induced by chemical allergens will result in the development of second generation predictive test methods in the mouse.

References

ASHBY, J., HILTON, J., DEARMAN, R.J., CALLANDER, R.D. and KIMBER, I., 1993. Mechanistic relationship among mutagenicity, skin sensitization and skin carcinogenicity. *Environmental Health Perspectives*, **101**, 62–7.

ASHERSON, G.L. and PTAK, W., 1968. Contact and delayed hypersensitivity in the mouse. I. Active sensitization and passive transfer. *Immunology*, **15**, 405–16.

BASKETTER, D.A. and SCHOLES, E.W., 1992. Comparison of the local lymph node assay with the guinea-pig maximization test for the detection of a range of contact allergens. *Food and Chemical Toxicology*, **60**, 65–9.

BASKETTER, D.A., SCHOLES, E.W., CUMBERBATCH, M., EVANS, C.D. and KIMBER, I., 1992. Sulphanilic acid: divergent results in the guinea pig maximization test and the local lymph node assay. *Contact Dermatitis*, **27**, 209–3.

BASKETTER, D.A., SCHOLES, E.W. and KIMBER, I., 1994. The performance of the local lymph node assay with chemicals identified as contact allergens in the human maximization test. *Food and Chemical Toxicology*, **32**, 543–7.

BASKETTER, D.A., SCHOLES, E.W., KIMBER, I., BOTHAM, P.A., HILTON, J., MILLER, K., ROBBINS, M.C., HARRISON, P.T.C. and WAITE, S.J., 1991. Interlaboratory evaluation of the local lymph node assay with 25 chemicals and comparison with guinea pig test data. *Toxicology Methods*, **1**, 30–43.

BASKETTER, D.A., SELBIE, E., SCHOLES, E.W., LEES, D., KIMBER, I. and BOTHAM, P.A., 1993. Results with OECD recommended positive control sensitizers in the maximization, Buehler and local lymph node assays. *Food and Chemical Toxicology*, **31**, 63–7.

BOTHAM, P.A., HILTON, J., EVANS, C.D., LEES, D. and HALL, T.J., 1991. Assessment of the relative skin sensitizing potency of 3 biocides using the murine local lymph node assay. *Contact Dermatitis*, **25**, 172–7.

CORNACOFF, J.B., HOUSE, R.V. and DEAN, J.H., 1988. Comparison of a radioisotopic incorporation method and the mouse ear swelling test (MEST) for contact sensitivity to weak sensitizers. *Fundamental and Applied Toxicology*, **10**, 40–4.

CUMBERBATCH, M., SCOTT, R.C., BASKETTER, D.A., SCHOLES, E.W., HILTON, J., DEARMAN, R.J. and KIMBER, I., 1993. Influence of sodium lauryl sulphate on 2,4-dinitrochlorobenzene-induced lymph node activation. *Toxicology*, **77**, 181–91.

DEARMAN, R.J., HOPE, J.C., HOPKINS, S.J., DEBICKI, R.J. and KIMBER, I., 1993. Interleukin 6 (IL-6) production by lymph node cells: an alternative endpoint for the local lymph node assay. *Toxicology Methods*, **3**, 268–78.

DEARMAN, R.J. and KIMBER, I., 1994. Cytokine production and the local lymph node assay, in Rougier, A., Goldberg, A.M. and Maibach, H.I. (eds), *In Vitro Skin Toxicology*, pp. 367–72, New York: Mary Ann Liebert.

DEARMAN, R.J., SCHOLES, E.W., RAMDIN, L.S.P., BASKETTER, D.A. and KIMBER, I., 1994. The local lymph node assay: an interlaboratory evaluation of interleukin 6 (IL-6) production by draining lymph node cells. *Journal of Applied Toxicology*, **14**, 287–91.

DESCOTES, J., 1988. Identification of contact allergens: the mouse ear sensitization assay. *Journal of Toxicology – Cutaneous and Ocular Toxicology*, **7**, 263–72.

DUNN, B.J., RUSCH, G.M., SIGLIN, J.C. and BLASZCAK, D.L., 1990. Variability of a mouse ear swelling test (MEST) in predicting weak and moderate contact sensitization. *Fundamental and Applied Toxicology*, **15**, 242–8.

EDWARDS, D.A., SORANNO, T.M., AMORUSO, M.A., HOUSE, R.V., TUMMEY, A.C., TRIMMER, G.W., THOMAS, P.T. and RIBEIRO, P.L., 1994. Screening petrochemicals for contact hypersensitivity potential: a comparison of the murine local lymph node assay with guinea pig and human test data. *Fundamental and Applied Toxicology*, **23**, 179–87.

EIPERT, E.F. and MILLER, H.C., 1975. Contact sensitivity in mice measured with thymidine labelled lymphocytes. *Immunological Communications*, **4**, 361–72.

GAD, S.C., 1994. The mouse ear swelling test (MEST) in the 1990s. *Toxicology*, **93**, 33–46.

GAD, S.C., DUNN, B.J., DOBBS, D.W., REILLY, C. and WALSH, R.D., 1986. Development and validation of an alternative dermal sensitization test: the mouse ear swelling test. *Toxicology and Applied Pharmacology*, **84**, 93–114.

GARRIGUE, J-L., NICOLAS, J-F., FRAGINALS, R., BENEZRA, C., BOUR, H. and SCHMITT, D., 1994. Optimization of the mouse ear swelling test for in vivo and in vitro studies of weak contact sensitizers. *Contact Dermatitis*, **30**, 231–7.

GERBERICK, G.F., HOUSE, R.V., FLETCHER, E.R. and RYAN, C.A., 1992. Examination of the local lymph node assay for use in contact sensitization risk assessment. *Fundamental and Applied Toxicology*, **19**, 438–45.

HILTON, J., DEARMAN, R.J., DEBICKI, R.J., RAMDIN, L.S.P. and KIMBER, I., 1994. Interleukin 6 production in vitro: an alternative read-out for the local lymph node assay. *Toxicology In Vitro*, **8**, 711–13.

HOPKINS, S.J., HUMPHREYS, M., KINNAIRD, A., JONES, D.A. and KIMBER, I., 1990. Production of interleukin-1 by draining lymph node cells during the induction phase of contact sensitization in mice. *Immunology*, **71**, 493–6.

HOPE, J.C., DEARMAN, R.J., KIMBER, I. and HOPKINS, S.J., 1994. The kinetics of cytokine production by draining lymph node cells following primary exposure of mice to chemical allergens. *Immunology*, **83**, 250–5.

IKARASHI Y., OHNO, K., MOMMA, J., TSUCHIYA, T. and NAKAMURA, A., 1994. Assessment of contact sensitivity of four thiourea rubber accelerators: comparison of two mouse lymph node assays with the guinea pig maximization test. *Food and Chemical Toxicology*, **32**, 1067–72.

IKARASHI Y., TSUCHIYA, T. and NAKAMURA, A., 1992. Detection of contact sensitivity of metal salts using the murine local lymph node assay. *Toxicology Letters*, **62**, 53–61.

1993a. Evaluation of contact sensitivity of rubber chemicals using the murine local lymph node assay. *Contact Dermatitis*, **28**, 77–80.

1993b. A sensitive mouse lymph node assay with two application phases for detection of contact allergens. *Archives of Toxicology*, **67**, 629–36.

IKARASHI Y., TSUKAMOTO, Y., TSUCHIYA, T. and NAKAMURA, A., 1993c. Influence of irritants on lymph node cell proliferation and the detection of contact sensitivity to metal salts in the murine local lymph node assay. *Contact Dermatitis*, **29**, 128–32.

KIMBER, I., 1989. Aspects of the immune response to contact allergens: opportunities for the development and modification of predictive test methods. *Food and Chemical Toxicology*, **27**, 755–62.

1992. Contact sensitivity, in Miller, K., Turk, J. and Nicklin, S. (eds), *Principles and Practice of Immunotoxicology*, pp. 104–24, Oxford: Blackwell.

1993. The murine local lymph node assay: principles and practice. *American Journal of Contact Dermatitis*, **4**, 42–4.

KIMBER, I. and BASKETTER, D.A., 1992. The murine local lymph node assay: a commentary on collaborative studies and new directions. *Food and Chemical Toxicology*, **30**, 165–9.

KIMBER, I., CUMBERBATCH, M. and COLEMAN, J.W., 1991a. Serum histamine and the elicitation of murine contact sensitivity. *Journal of Applied Toxicology*, **11**, 339–42.

KIMBER, I., CUMBERBATCH, M., HUMPHREYS, M. and HOPKINS, S.J., 1990a. Contact hypersensitivity induces plasma interleukin 6. *International Archives of Allergy and Applied Immunology*, **92**, 97–9.

KIMBER, I. and DEARMAN, R.J., 1991. Investigation of lymph node cell proliferation as a possible immunological correlate of contact sensitizing potential. *Food and Chemical Toxicology*, **29**, 125–9.

1993. Approaches to the identification and classification of chemical allergens in mice. *Journal of Pharmacological and Toxicological Methods*, **29**, 11–16.

1994. Assessment of contact and respiratory sensitivity in mice, in Dean, J.H., Luster, M.I., Munson, A.E. and Kimber, I. (eds), *Immunotoxicology and Immunopharmacology*, pp. 721–32, New York: Raven Press.

KIMBER, I., DEARMAN, R.J., SCHOLES, E.W. and BASKETTER, D.A., 1994. The local lymph node assay: developments and applications. *Toxicology*, **93**, 13–31.

KIMBER, I., GERBERICK, G.F., VAN LOVEREN, H. and HOUSE, R.V., 1992. Chemical allergy: molecular mechanisms and practical applications. *Fundamental and Applied Toxicology*, **19**, 479–83.

KIMBER, I., HILTON, J. and BOTHAM, P.A., 1990b. Identification of contact allergens using the murine local lymph node assay: comparisons with the Buehler occluded patch test in guinea pigs. *Journal of Applied Toxicology*, **10**, 173–80.

KIMBER, I., HILTON, J., BOTHAM, P.A., BASKETTER, D.A., SCHOLES, E.W., MILLER, K., ROBBINS, M.C., HARRISON, P.T.C., GRAY, T.J.B. and WAITE, S.J., 1991b. The murine local lymph node assay: results of an interlaboratory trial. *Toxicology Letters*, **55**, 203–13.

KIMBER, I., HILTON, J., DEARMAN, R.J., GERBERICK, G.F., RYAN, C.A., BASKETTER, D.A., SCHOLES, E.W., LADICS, G.S., LOVELESS, S.E., HOUSE, R.V. and GUY, A., 1995. An international evaluation of the murine local lymph node assay and comparison of modified procedures. *Toxicology*, in press.

KIMBER, I., HILTON, J. and WEISENBERGER, C., 1989a. The murine local lymph node assay for identification of contact allergens: a preliminary evaluation of in situ measurement of lymphocyte proliferation. *Contact Dermatitis*, **21**, 215–20.

KIMBER, I., MITCHELL, J.A. and GRIFFIN, A.C., 1986. Development of a murine local lymph node assay for the determination of sensitizing potential. *Food and Chemical Toxicology*, **24**, 585–6.

KIMBER, I., SHEPHERD, C.J., MITCHELL, J.A., TURK, J.L. and BAKER, D., 1989b. Regulation of lymphocyte proliferation in contact sensitivity: homeostatic mechanisms and a possible explanation of antigenic competition. *Immunology*, **66**, 577–82.

KIMBER, I., WARD, R.K., SHEPHERD, C.J., SMITH, M.N., McADAM, K.P.W.J. and RAYNES, J.G., 1989c. Acute-phase proteins and serological evaluation of experimental contact sensitivity in the mouse. *International Archives of Allergy and Applied Immunology*, **89**, 149–55.

KIMBER, I. and WEISENBERGER, C., 1989a. A murine local lymph node assay for the identification of contact allergens. Assay development and results of an initial validation study. *Archives of Toxicology*, **63**, 274–82.

1989b. A modified local lymph node assay for identification of contact allergens, in Frosch, P.J., Dooms-Goossens, A., Lachapelle, J-M., Rycroft, R.J.G. and Scheper, R.J. (eds), *Current Topics in Contact Dermatitis*, pp. 592–5, Heidelberg: Springer-Verlag.

1991. Anamnestic responses to contact allergens: applications in the murine local lymph node assay. *Journal of Applied Toxicology*, **11**, 129–33.

MAISEY, J. and MILLER, K., 1986. Assessment of the ability of mice fed on vitamin A supplemented diet to respond to a variety of potential contact sensitizers. *Contact Dermatitis*, **15**, 17–23.

MALKOVSKY, M., DORE, C., HUNT, R., PALMER, L., CHANDLER, P. and MEDAWAR, P.B., 1983a. Enhancement of specific antitumor immunity in mice fed a diet enriched in vitamin A acetate. *Proceedings of the National Academy of Sciences, USA*, **80**, 6322–6.

MALKOVSKY, M., EDWARDS, A.J., HUNT, R., PALMER, L. and MEDAWAR, P.B., 1983b. T-cell-mediated enhancement of host-versus-graft reactivity in mice fed a diet enriched in vitamin A acetate. *Nature, London*, **302**, 338–40.

MARCINKEIWICZ, J. and CHAIN, B.M., 1989. Antigen-specific inhibition of IL-2 and IL-3 production in contact sensitivity to TNP. *Immunology*, **68**, 185–92.

1990. Further studies on the regulation of lymphokine biosynthesis in contact sensitivity. *Cytokine*, **2**, 344–52.

MEKORI, Y.A., DVORAK, H.F. and GALLI, S.J., 1986. ^{125}I-fibrin deposition in contact sensitivity reactions in the mouse. Sensitivity of the assay for quantitating reactions after active or passive sensitization. *Journal of Immunology*, **136**, 2018–25.

MILLER, K., MAISEY, J. and MALKOVSKY, M., 1984. Enhancement of contact sensitization in mice fed a diet enriched in vitamin A acetate. *International Archives of Allergy and Applied Immunology*, **75**, 120–5.

MONTELIUS, J., WAHLKVIST, H., BOMAN, A., FERNSTROM, P., GRABERGS, L. and WAHLBERG, J.E., 1994. Experience with the murine local lymph node assay: inability to discriminate between allergens and irritants. *Acta Dermatology Venereology*, **74**, 22–7.

OECD (Organization for Economic Cooperation and Development), 1992. *Guideline 406 for Testing Chemicals*. Adopted 1992.

OLIVER, G.J.A., BOTHAM, P.A. and KIMBER, I., 1986. Models for contact sensitization – novel approaches and future developments. *British Journal of Dermatology*, **115**, (Suppl. 31) 53–62.

PFENNIG, K. and ZIEGLER, V., 1991. Detection of allergens by lymph node assay. *Zeitschrift fuer Hautkrankheiten*, **66**, 959–63.

POTTER, D.W. and HAZELTON, G.A., 1995. Evaluation of auricular lymph node cell proliferation in isothiazolone-treated mice. *Fundamental and Applied Toxicology*, **24**, 165–72.

RODENBERGER, S.L., LEDGER, P.W. and PREVO, M.E., 1993. Murine model for contact sensitization. *Toxicology Methods*, **3**, 157–68.

SABBADINI, E., NERI, A. and SEHON, A.H., 1974. Localisation of non-immune radioactively labelled cells in the lesions of contact sensitivity in mice. *Journal of Immunological Methods*, **5**, 9–19.

SAILSTAD, D.M., KRISHNAN, S.D., TEPPER, J.S., DOERFLER, D.L. and SELGRADE, M.K., 1995. Dietary vitamin A enhances sensitivity of the local lymph node assay. *Toxicology*, **96**, 157–63.

SAILSTAD, D.M., TEPPER, J.S., DOERFLER, D.L., QASIM, M. and SELGRADE, M.K., 1994. Evaluation of an azo and two anthraquinone dyes for allergic potential. *Fundamental and Applied Toxicology*, **23**, 569–77.

SAILSTAD, D.M., TEPPER, J.S., DOERFLER, D.L. and SELGRADE, M.K., 1993. Evaluation of several variations of the mouse ear swelling test (MEST) for detection of weak and moderate contact sensitizers. *Toxicology Methods*, **3**, 169–82.

SCHOLES, E.W., BASKETTER, D.A., SARLL, A.E., KIMBER, I., EVANS, C.D., MILLER, K., ROBBINS, M.C., HARRISON, P.T.C. and WAITE, S.J., 1992. The local lymph node assay: results of a final inter-laboratory validation under field conditions. *Journal of Applied Toxicology*, **12**, 217–22.

STRINGER, C.P., HICKS, R. and BOTHAM, P.A., 1991. Contact sensitivity (allergic contact dermatitis) to bis(tri-n-butyltin) oxide in mice. *Contact Dermatitis*, **24**, 210–5.

THORNE, P.S., HAWK, C., KALISZEWSKI, S.D. and GUINEY, P.D., 1991a. The noninvasive mouse ear swelling assay. I. Refinements for detecting weak sensitizers. *Fundamental and Applied Toxicology*, **17**, 790–806.

1991b. The noninvasive mouse ear swelling assay. II. Testing the contact sensitizing potency of fragrances. *Fundamental and Applied Toxicology*, **17**, 807–20.

9

Alternative Methods for Contact Sensitization Testing

I. KIMBER

Zeneca Central Toxicology Laboratory, Macclesfield

Introduction

In common with other areas of toxicology, there is presently considerable interest in the possibility of developing alternative methods for contact sensitizing testing that have a reduced requirement for experimental animals, that reduce the trauma to which animals are potentially subject, or that eliminate completely the need for animals. As described in the previous chapter, much progress has been made already in defining mouse predictive tests which offer advantages with respect to animal numbers and/or potential trauma. There are, however, additional initiatives and approaches and some of these are discussed below. The objective ultimately is the accurate identification and characterization of skin sensitizing chemicals without the need for animal experimentation. Within this context one can identify two main strategies. Firstly, there is the use of structure-activity relationships (SAR), or quantitative structure-activity relationships (QSAR), linked to the development of expert, rule-based, systems (Barratt *et al.*, 1994, Barratt and Basketter, 1994). This area is explored in detail in Chapter 5. The second approach is the use in predictive toxicology of *in vitro* models that mirror accurately some important aspect of the skin sensitization process. The goal is laudable; the difficulty of achieving it, however, should not be under-estimated. The primary constraints in developing workable models of immune function *in vitro* are the complexity of the immune system itself, and the requirement of normal immunological activity for complex interactions between cells and molecules that are tightly coordinated and regulated in time and space. Notwithstanding these difficulties, advances have been made in the design of alternative methods and these are described here under

140

headings that reflect the main areas of activity: allergen-driven T lymphocyte activation, the stimulation of epidermal cell responses and the association of chemical allergens with protein.

Measurement of T Lymphocyte Activation

As described in Chapter 2, the central event during the induction phase of skin sensitization is the stimulation in draining lymph nodes of T lymphocyte activation. Measurement of induced T lymphocyte proliferative responses, either *in situ* or *in vitro* forms the basis of the local lymph node assay (Chapter 8). Antigen-driven T cell activation can be modelled *in vitro* if responsive T lymphocytes are cultured with antigen in a suitable form and with an appropriate source of antigen presenting and/or accessory cells. Thus, lymphocytes isolated from contact sensitized mice will mount secondary proliferative responses *in vitro* when cultured under correct conditions with the inducing chemical allergen (Phanuphak *et al.*, 1974; Kimber *et al.*, 1986). The phenomenon forms the basis of the lymphocyte transformation test (LTT), a method used for the investigation of allergic contact dermatitis in man. The potential value of the LTT is that it may provide a method whereby the causative allergen can be identified without the need for diagnostic patch testing (von Blomberg-van der Flier *et al.*, 1989). The majority of studies has focused on nickel allergy where it has been found that peripheral blood mononuclear cells isolated from nickel-sensitive, but not control (non-sensitized), donors will mount proliferative responses when cultured with an appropriate concentration of nickel sulphate or chloride (Macleod *et al.*, 1970; Hutchinson *et al.*, 1972; Al-Tawil *et al.*, 1981; von Blomberg-van der Flier *et al.*, 1987; Everness *et al.*, 1990; Kimber *et al.*, 1990). The stimulation of responses in the LTT by lipophilic allergens that will not dissolve readily in aqueous solutions is less straightforward. One approach that has proved successful is the use of conjugates formed between the chemical hapten and an immunologically inert protein, such as (in man) human serum albumin (Kimber *et al.*, 1991). Some of the chemical allergens investigated using the human lymphocyte transformation test are listed in Table 9.1.

Lymphocyte blastogenesis tests in mice, or less commonly in guinea pigs, have been used, either as independent assays or in association with other methods, for toxicological evaluation (Robinson, 1989; Robinson and Sneller, 1990; Gerberick *et al.*, 1990, 1991; Kashima *et al.*, 1993; Nicolas *et al.*, 1994). In the examples cited above measurement is made of secondary T lymphocyte proliferative responses stimulated by allergen in cells isolated from previously sensitized animals. An intriguing question is whether it is possible also to provoke *in vitro* primary allergen-specific responses by lymphocytes prepared from naive animals (or humans). Unprimed (virgin) T lymphocytes and memory cells that are the progeny of a proliferative response resulting from previous encounter with antigen may be distin-

Table 9.1 Human lymphocyte transformation test

Allergen tested	Reference
Nickel	Macleod *et al.*, 1970; Hutchinson *et al.*, 1972; Al-Tawil *et al.*, 1981; von Blomberg van der Flier *et al.*, 1987; Everness *et al.*, 1990; Kimber *et al.*, 1990
Neomycin sulphate	Kimber *et al.*, 1990
Chromium	Yamada *et al.*, 1972
2,4-Dinitrochlorobenzene (DNCB)	Miller and Levis, 1973; Soeberg and Anderson, 1976; Levis *et al.*, 1976; Kimber *et al.*, 1990
Urushiol	Byers *et al.*, 1979
Thiurams	Kimber *et al.*, 1991

guished phenotypically as a function of CD45 isoform expression. As discussed in Chapter 2, memory cells display a truncated form of the molecule, designated CD45RO, while virgin T lymphocytes are characterized by possession of the high molecular weight isoform, CD45RA (Akbar *et al.*, 1988). These populations differ also in their need for antigen presentation. The requirements for the initial antigen-driven activation of virgin T lymphocytes are more rigorous than those necessary for the restimulation of memory cells (Gajewski *et al.*, 1989; Metlay *et al.*, 1989). The differential activation thresholds for unprimed and memory T lymphocytes translate into a variable dependency upon antigen-presenting cells. A variety of antigen presenting cell populations, including 'non-professional' antigen presenting cells, is able to effect the restimulation of memory T lymphocytes. However, dendritic cells are necessary for the activation of virgin T lymphocytes (Inaba and Steinman, 1984). There is no doubt that, on a per cell basis, dendritic cells are considerably more active than are other populations in stimulating secondary T lymphocyte responses *in vitro*. As a consequence, in most of the mouse blastogenesis assays quoted above, antigen-bearing dendritic cells isolated from the lymph nodes of sensitized animals or hapten-modified Langerhans cell (LC)-enriched epidermal cells have proved most effective at stimulating proliferative responses by primed T lymphocytes. The question is whether such populations have the capacity also to induce primary T cell responses to chemical allergens *in vitro*. There is evidence that this is in fact the case. It has been shown that antigen-bearing dendritic cells enriched from the draining lymph nodes of previously sensitized mice will provoke *in vitro* proliferative responses by T lymphocytes prepared from naive syngeneic donors (Knight *et al.*, 1985; Macatonia *et al.*, 1986). A detailed analysis of induced primary proliferative responses *in vitro* was performed by Hauser and Katz (1988) in which the ability of hapten-modified LC to activate T lymphocytes from naive mice was examined. In these studies autoreactive T cells activated by culture with normal syngeneic LC were eliminated by treatment with bromodeoxyuridine and light. The residual population of T lymphocytes was shown to be only minimally responsive to culture with normal LC, but to mount a vigorous proliferative response when mixed with hapten-modified LC. In the same series of experiments the specificity of induced primary responses was examined. Prior removal of T cells responsive to one hapten did not impair restimulation *in vitro* by LC modified with a second, unrelated chemical allergen (Hauser and Katz, 1988).

Attempts have been made to capitalize upon these observations, the objective being to provoke specific T lymphocyte responses using only responder populations from naive mice or unsensitized humans. If successful such an approach would obviate the need for active sensitization. Moulon *et al.* (1993, 1994) have shown that human epidermal LC modified *in vitro* with the trinitrophenyl (TNP) hapten (the haptenic moiety deriving from the potent contact allergen, trinitrochlorobenzene) will provoke in autologous peripheral blood T cells a significant proliferative response. Similar results were obtained when responder T lymphocyte populations were enriched for cells expressing CD45RA, confirming that the responses observed were due primarily to the activation of naive cells (Moulon *et al.*, 1993). Consistent with the fact that freshly isolated LC are comparatively ineffective antigen presenting cells (Schuler and Steinman, 1985; see Chapter 2), it was found that primary responses were provoked only if the stimulator cells had first been cultured to achieve functional maturation (Moulon *et al.*, 1993). While the data reviewed above are encouraging, insofar as they demonstrate that, in principle, it is possible to explore *in vitro* whether a chemical is likely to stimulate specific T cell responses, it must be remembered that to date only a very limited number of potent contact allergens has been shown to be active. It remains to be determined whether a wide range of skin sensitizers is able to induce the activation of virgin allergen-responsive T cells *in vitro*.

Epidermal Responses and Cytokine Production

The skin is, by definition, the route of exposure for contact sensitization. As discussed in detail in Chapter 2, the skin is an immunologically active tissue and epidermal cells produce constitutively or can be stimulated to produce a variety of cytokines (Kimber, 1993; Cumberbatch and Kimber, 1994). Many of these cytokines play important roles in the regulation of LC movement and function and some at least are required for the optimal induction of skin sensitization (Chapter 2). It is not surprising therefore that there exists considerable interest in determining whether chemical allergens can be identified as a function of induced epidermal cell cytokine production and whether, on the same basis, sensitizers can be distinguished from cutaneous irritants. Clearly the expectation is that if contact allergens provoke a characteristic pattern of epidermal cytokine expression then this would pave the way toward an *in vitro* predictive method using skin explants or cultured cells.

It is apparent that some epidermal cytokines will be induced or upregulated by a variety of stimuli. For example, the production by keratinocytes of tumour necrosis factor α (TNF-α) is increased following topical exposure to chemical allergens, the application of skin irritants or in response to ultraviolet B irradiation (Kock *et al.*, 1990; Enk and Katz, 1992a, c). Nevertheless, there have been suggestions that the induction or increased expression of some other skin cytokines may be a selective property of chemical allergens. Using a reverse-transcriptase polymerase chain reaction (PCR) technique, Enk and Katz (1992a, b, c) examined changes in the expression of mRNA for a variety of epidermal cytokines following exposure of mice to chemical allergens such as 2,4-dinitrofluorobenzene (DNFB), or to a non-sensitizing skin irritant, sodium lauryl sulphate (SLS). They reported that while both allergens and irritants stimulated the increased expression of mRNA for certain epidermal cytokines, such as TNF-α, granulocyte/macrophage colony-stimulating factor (GM-CSF) and interferon-γ (IFN-γ), the latter being a product of infiltrating T lymphocytes, only skin sensitizing chemicals upregulated interleukins 1 α and β (IL-1α and IL-1β), interleukin 10 (IL-10), IFN-induced protein 10 (IP-10) and macrophage inflammatory protein 2 (MIP-2). Moreover, the expression by LC of mRNA for major histocompatibility complex class II (Ia) antigens was increased only by exposure to chemical allergens. These observations are intriguing, but require confirmation with a wider range of allergens and skin irritants. In addition, it is not certain that even if such selective patterns can be reproducibly stimulated *in vivo*, they will necessarily be mirrored across species and by changes induced *in vitro*. Using cultures of human keratinocytes Wilmer *et al.* (1994) found that several skin irritants, including croton oil, phenol and benzalkonium chloride, each induced an increase in intracellular IL-1α, a cytokine suggested from the studies of Enk and Katz (1992a, c) to be upregulated only by allergens. Also using cultured human keratinocytes it was demonstrated by Pastore *et al.* (1995) in a separate investigation that skin sensitizers had variable effects on the expression of IL-1α mRNA. Although neomycin sulphate caused a dose-dependent increase in mRNA for IL-1α, benzocaine was without effect and dinitro-benzene sulphonate suppressed IL-1α gene expression.

Despite some uncertainty, the prospect of identifying skin allergens as a function of epidermal cytokine production *in vitro* remains an objective. The models selected for such studies include the use of cultured keratinocytes (Pastore *et al.*, 1995) or three-dimensional skin equivalents comprising dermal fibroblasts and keratinocytes (Harvell *et al.*, 1994; De Wever and Rheins, 1994). The use of such models, in the context of characterizing induced changes in epidermal cytokine expression may, however, be subject to one important limitation – the absence of Langerhans cells. In recent years it has become apparent that LC produce certain cytokines. In fact, for some cytokines LC may represent the exclusive, or at least most important, source within the epidermis. It has been shown, for instance, on the basis of mRNA expression, that within murine epidermis LC represent the sole source of constitutive or allergen-induced IL-1β (Enk and Katz, 1992a; Schreiber *et al.*, 1992; Matsue *et al.*, 1992; Heufler *et al.*, 1992). Furthermore, macrophage inflammatory protein 1α (MIP-1α) in the mouse epidermis derives largely or wholly from LC (Matsue *et al.*, 1992; Heufler *et al.*, 1992) and LC appear to be an important, although not exclusive, source of interleukin 6 (IL-6) (Schreiber *et al.*, 1992). The fact that one of the cytokines suggested by the studies of Enk and Katz (1992a, c) to be upregulated selectively by chemical allergens is produced only by LC serves to emphasize the importance of these cells in the epidermal cytokine network and the need to consider their contribution when examining responses induced in the skin by chemicals.

It may prove that IL-1β is a particularly relevant molecular marker of skin sensitization. Not only is the expression of IL-1β by LC increased following topical exposure to contact allergens, it appears that the availability of sufficient quantities of this cytokine is required for optimal induction of cutaneous immune responses (Enk *et al.*, 1993). If one speculates that the stimulation of IL-1β production during skin sensitization results from the direct interaction of the chemical allergen with resident LC, which may be the case (Trede *et al.*, 1991), then it can be argued that this might provide the basis for an alternative approach to characterization *in vitro* of allergenic potential using purified LC. In practice the major problem that presents itself is the availability of cells. Langerhans cells within the epidermis and related dendritic cells in other tissues represent always minority populations and isolation, on a routine basis, of sufficient cells for *in vitro* analyses would undoubtedly prove difficult. A possible solution may be provided by the demonstration recently that the cytokines TNF-α and GM-CSF act in concert to drive the development *in vitro* of dendritic cells from CD34[+] haemopoietic progenitors (Inaba *et al.*, 1992; Santiago-Schwarz *et al.*, 1992; Caux *et al.*, 1992).

Further experimentation may indicate that the identification and characterization of cutaneous toxicants on the basis simply of qualitative changes in epidermal cytokine expression may not be realistic. The induction and/or upregulation of cytokine production in the skin is complex and dependent upon both the nature and severity of the external stimulus and local immunoregulatory events such as the autocrine and paracrine influences of cytokines themselves. Consequently, different forms of skin insult may be reflected more accurately by the vigour and tempo of induced changes in epidermal cytokine expression. Until there is confirmation that chemical allergens induce in skin selective cytokine expression patterns it is worth considering whether it may be possible presently to approach the issue in a different way and to identify chemicals that are unlikely to cause skin sensitization. Certain epidermal cytokines are essential for skin sensitization, or at least for the optimal induction of sensitization. Treatment of mice with neutralizing antibodies for IL-1β and TNF-α inhibits or impairs the development of contact sensitization (Enk *et al.*, 1993; Cumberbatch and Kimber, 1995), the implication being that chemicals that fail to cause the increased expression of these cytokines will also fail to induce sensitization. The value of such an approach in the initial assessment of chemicals remains unexplored.

One other aspect of epidermal cell responses during skin sensitization is worthy of consideration. Topical exposure of mice to chemical allergens has been reported to result in the activation of LC and the stimulation of absorptive endocytosis. Similar treatment with non-sensitizing skin irritants results only in degenerative changes in local LC (Kolde and Knop, 1987). There is other evidence that contact allergens will induce in resident LC phenotypic and functional changes. Aiba and Katz (1990) observed that exposure of mice to chemical allergens, but not to SLS, caused a substantial increase in the membrane expression of Ia antigen by a proportion of LC. Consistent with this is the fact that skin sensitizers stimulate the increased expression by epidermal cells of mRNA for this determinant (Enk and Katz, 1992a). Chemical sensitizers may influence the localization as well as level of expression of Ia antigens by LC. The allergen DNFB has been found to induce the internalization of Ia molecules, a process that may be essential for the efficient processing of antigen by LC (Becker *et al.*, 1992a,b). Similarly, there are reports that treatment of epidermal cells with sensitizing agents results in an activation of LC that is characterized by the presence of rough endoplasmic reticulum and numerous endocytic vesicles (Picut *et al.*, 1987; Barbier *et al.*, 1994). The opportunities that may exist for the development of *in vitro* predictive tests based upon the changes induced in LC by chemical allergens are being explored currently within the context of an interlaboratory collaboration (Barbier *et al.*, 1994).

Association with Protein

Chemical allergens are haptens and as such are unable to stimulate directly an immune response. The realization of immunogenicity is dependent upon their association with protein to form a hapten conjugate. There exists therefore a correlation between protein reactivity, or protein reactivity achieved following local biotransformation, and skin sensitization potential (Dupuis and Benezra, 1981; Basketter and Roberts, 1990). A prospective screen for sensitizing activity could include an assessment *in vitro* of the ability of test materials to form covalent associations with a defined protein or peptide. One example serves to illustrate the point. It has been proposed that evaluation of protein reactivity should form part of a tiered approach to the identification of chemical respiratory allergens, the method selected being measurement of the association of test materials with albumin using high performance liquid chromatography (Sarlo and Clark, 1992; Gauggel *et al.*, 1993). Although the above was developed specifically for investigation of respiratory sensitization potential, the principles apply equally to contact allergy. While measurement of association with protein *in vitro* may be useful in eliminating those chemicals that are unlikely to form stable immunogenic conjugates *in vivo*, it must be borne in mind that some agents will require metabolic activation to a reactive species. Equally important is the fact that the formation of strong covalent complexes with protein does not of itself guarantee sensitizing activity. As discussed in Chapter 2, for the effective induction of skin sensitization a chemical must be able to penetrate into the viable skin across the stratum corneum. It will be necessary therefore to consider lipophilicity and skin permeability alongside estimates of inherent or inducible protein reactivity.

Conclusion

Advances have been made. However, there are at present no methods that could be regarded as true *in vitro* alternatives to standard predictive tests. Undoubtedly new opportunities will arise from a more detailed understanding of the complex biological events triggered by exposure to skin sensitizing chemicals and the way in which those events differ from changes caused by other types of cutaneous toxicant.

References

AIBA, S. and KATZ, S.I., 1990, Phenotypic and functional characteristics of in vivo-activated Langerhans cells, *Journal of Immunology*, **145**, 2791–6.

AKBAR, A.N., TERRY, L., TIMMS, A., BEVERLEY, P.C.L. and JANOSSY, G., 1988, Loss of CD45R and gain of UCHL1 reactivity is a feature of primed T cells, *Journal of Immunology*, **140**, 2171–8.

AL-TAWIL, N.G., MARCUSSON, J.A. and MOLLER, E., 1981, Lymphocyte transformation test in patients with nickel sensitivity: an aid to diagnosis, *Archives Dermatology Venereology*, **61**, 511–5.

BARBIER, A., RIZOVA, E., STAMPF, J.L., LACHERETZ, F., PISTOOR, F.H.M., BOS, J.D., KAPSENBERG, M.L., BECKER, D., MOHAMADZADEH, M., KNOP, J., MABIC, S. and LEPOITTEVIN, J-P., 1994, Development of a predictive in vitro test for detection of sensitizing compounds (European Bridge Project), in Rougier, A., Goldberg, A.M. and Maibach, H.I. (eds), *In Vitro Skin Toxicology, Irritation, Phototoxicity, Sensitization*, pp. 341–50, New York: Mary Ann Liebert.

BARRATT, M.D. and BASKETTER, D.A., 1994, Structure-activity relationships for skin sensitization: an expert system, in Rougier, A., Goldberg, A.M. and Maibach, H.I., (eds), *In Vitro Skin Toxicology, Irritation, Phototoxicity, Sensitization*, pp. 293–301, New York: Mary Ann Liebert.

BARRATT, M.D., BASKETTER, D.A., CHAMBERLAIN, M., PAYNE, M.P., ADAMS, G. and LANGOWSKI, J., 1994, Development of an expert system rulebase for identifying contact allergens, *Toxicology in Vitro*, **8**, 837–9.

BASKETTER, D.A. and ROBERTS, D.W., 1990, A quantitative structure activity/dose relationship for contact allergic potential of alkyl transfer agents, *Toxicology In Vitro*, **4**, 686–7.

BECKER, D., MOHAMADZADEH, M., RESKE, K. and KNOP, J., 1992a, Increased level of intracellular MHC class II molecules in murine Langerhans cells following in vivo and in vitro administration of contact allergens, *Journal of Investigative Dermatology*, **99**, 545–9.

BECKER, D., NEISS, U., NEISS, S., RESKE, and KNOP, J., 1992b, Contact allergens modulate the expression of MHC class II molecules on murine epidermal Langerhans cells by endocytic mechanisms, *Journal of Investigative Dermatology*, **98**, 700–5.

BYERS, V.S., EPSTEIN, W.L., CASTAGNOLI, N. and BAER, H., 1979, In vitro studies of poison oak immunity. I. In vitro reaction of human lymphocytes to urushiol, *Journal of Clinical Investigation*, **64**, 1437–48.

CAUX, C., DEZUTTER-DAMBUYANT, C., SCHMITT, D. and BANCHEREAU, J., 1992, GM-CSF and TNF-α cooperate in the generation of dendritic Langerhans cells, *Nature*, **360**, 258–61.

CUMBERBATCH, M. and KIMBER, I., 1994, Epidermal cytokines and skin sensitization hazard, *Toxicology in Vitro*, **8**, 685–7.

1995, Tumour necrosis factor-α is required for accumulation of dendritic cells in draining lymph nodes and for optimal contact sensitization, *Immunology*, **84**, 31–5.

DE WEVER, B. and RHEINS, L.A., 1994, Skin^{2TM}. An in vitro human skin analog, in Rougier, A., Goldberg, A.M. and Maibach, H.I. (eds), *In Vitro Skin Toxicology, Irritation, Phototoxicity, Sensitization*, pp. 121–31, New York: Mary Ann Liebert.

DUPUIS, G. and BENEZRA, C., 1982, *Contact Dermatitis to Simple Chemicals: A Molecular Approach*, New York: Marcel Dekker.

ENK, A.H., ANGELONI, V.L., UDEY, M.C. and KATZ, S.I., 1993, An essential role for Langerhans cell-derived IL-1β in the initiation of primary immune responses in skin, *Journal of Immunology*, **150**, 3698–704.

ENK, A.H. and KATZ, S.I., 1992a, Early molecular events in the induction phase of contact sensitivity, *Proceedings of the National Academy of Sciences, USA*, **89**, 1398–402.

1992b, Identification and induction of keratinocyte-derived IL-10, *Journal of Immunology*, **149**, 92–5.

1992c, Early events in the induction phase of contact sensitivity, *Journal of Investigative Dermatology*, **99**, 39S–41S.

EVERNESS, K.M., GAWKRODGER, D.J., BOTHAM, P.A. and HUNTER, J.A.A., 1990, The discrimination between nickel-sensitive and non-nickel-sensitive subjects by an in vitro lymphocyte transformation test, *British Journal of Dermatology*, **122**, 293–8.

GAJEWSKI, T.F., SCHELL, S.R., NAU, G. and FITCH, F.W., 1989, Regulation of T cell activation: differences among T-cell subsets, *Immunological Reviews*, **111**, 79–110.

GAUGGEL, D.L., SARLO, K. and ASQUITH, T.N., 1993, A proposed screen for

148

evaluating low-molecular-weight chemicals as potential respiratory allergens, *Journal of Applied Toxicology*, **13**, 307–13.

GERBERICK, G.F., RYAN, C.A., FLETCHER, E.R., SNELLER, D.L. and ROBIN-SON, M.K., 1990, An optimized lymphocyte blastogenesis assay for detecting the response of contact sensitized or photosensitized lymphocytes to hapten or photohapten modified antigen presenting cells, *Toxicology in Vitro*, **4**, 289–92.

GERBERICK, G.F., RYAN, C.A., VON BARGEN, E.C., STUARD, S.B. and RIDDER, G.M., 1991, Examination of tetrachlorosalicylanilide (TCSA) photoallergy using in vitro photohapten-modified Langerhans cell-enriched epidermal cells, *Journal of Investigative Dermatology*, **97**, 210–8.

HARVELL, J.D., GAY, R. and MAIBACH, H.I., 1994, The living skin equivalent in cutaneous irritancy assessment, in Rougier, A., Goldberg, A.M. and Maibach, H.I. (eds), *In Vitro Skin Toxicology, Irritation, Phototoxicity, Sensitization*, pp. 117–9, New York: Mary Ann Liebert.

HAUSER, C. and KATZ, S.I., 1988, Activation and expansion of hapten- and protein-specific T-helper cells from non-sensitized mice, *Proceedings of the National Academy of Sciences, USA*, **85**, 5625–8.

HEUFLER, C., TOPAR, G., KOCH, F., TROCKENBACHER, B., KAMPGEN, E., ROMANI, N. and SCHULER, G., 1992, Cytokine gene expression in murine epidermal cell suspensions: interleukin 1β and macrophage inflammatory protein 1α are selectively expressed in Langerhans cells but are differently regulated in culture, *Journal of Experimental Medicine*, **176**, 1221–6.

HUTCHINSON, F., RAFFLE, E.J. and MACLEOD, T.M., 1972, The specificity of lymphocyte transformation in vitro by nickel salts in nickel sensitive subjects, *Journal of Investigative Dermatology*, **58**, 362–5.

INABA, K., INABA, M., ROMANI, N., AYA, H., DEGUCHI, M., IKERHARA, S., MURAMATSU, S. and STEINMAN, R.M., 1992, Generation of large numbers of dendritic cells from mouse bone marrow cultures supplemented with granulocyte/macrophage colony-stimulating factor, *Journal of Experimental Medicine*, **176**, 1693–702.

INABA, K. and STEINMAN, R.M., 1984, Resting and sensitized T lymphocytes exhibit distinct (antigen presenting cell) requirements for growth and lymphokine release, *Journal of Experimental Medicine*, **160**, 1717–35.

KASHIMA, R., OKADA, J., IKEDA, Y. and YOSHIZUKA, N., 1993, Challenge assay in vitro using lymphocyte blastogenesis for the contact hypersensivity assay, *Food and Chemical Toxicology*, **31**, 759–66.

KIMBER, I., 1993, Epidermal cytokines in contact hypersensitivity: immunological roles and practical applications, *Toxicology in Vitro*, **7**, 295–8.

KIMBER, I., BOTHAM, P.A., RATTRAY, N.J. and WALSH, S.J., 1986, Contact sensitizing and tolerogenic properties of 2,4-dinitrothiocyanobenzene, *International Archives of Allergy and Applied Immunology*, **81**, 258–64.

KIMBER, I., QUIRKE, S. and BECK, M.H., 1990, Attempts to identify the causative allergen in cases of allergic contact dermatitis using an in vitro lymphocyte transformation test, *Toxicology in Vitro*, **4**, 302–6.

KIMBER, I., QUIRKE, S., CUMBERBATCH, M., ASHBY, J., PATON, D., ALDRIDGE, R.D., HUNTER, J.A.A. and BECK, M.H., 1991, Lymphocyte transformation and thiuram sensitization, *Contact Dermatitis*, **24**, 164–71.

KNIGHT, S.C., KREJCI, J., MALKOVSKY, M., COLIZZI, V., GAUTAM, A. and ASHERSON, G.L., 1985, The role of dendritic cells in the initiation of immune responses to contact sensitizers. I. In vivo exposure to antigen, *Cellular Immunology*, **94**, 427–34.

KOCK, A., SCHWARZ, T., KIRNBAUER, R., URBANSKI, A., PERRY, P., ANSEL, J.C. and LUGER, T.A., 1990, Human keratinocytes are a source for human tumor necrosis factor α: evidence for synthesis and release upon stimulation with endotoxin or ultraviolet light, *Journal of Experimental Medicine*, **172**, 1609–14.

KOLDE, G. and KNOP, J., 1987, Different cellular reaction patterns of epidermal Langerhans cells after application of contact sensitizing, toxic and tolerogenic compounds. A comparative ultrastructural and morphometric time-course analysis, *Journal of Investigative Dermatology*, **89**, 19–23.

LEVIS, W.R., WHALEN, J.J. and POWELL, J.A., 1976, Specific blastogenesis and lymphokine production in DNCB-sensitive human leukocyte cultures stimulated with soluble and particulate DNP-containing antigens, *Clinical and Experimental Immunology*, **23**, 481–90.

MACATONIA, S.E., EDWARDS, A.J. and KNIGHT, S.C., 1986, Dendritic cells and the initiation of contact sensitivity to fluorescein isothiocyanate, *Immunology*, **59**, 509–14.

MACLEOD, T.M., HUTCHINSON, F. and RAFFLE, E.J., 1970, The uptake of labelled thymidine by leukocytes of nickel sensitive patients, *British Journal of Dermatology*, **82**, 487–92.

MATSUE, H., CRUZ, P.D. Jr., BERGSTRESSER, P.R. and TAKASHIMA, A., 1992, Langerhans cells are the major source of mRNA for IL-1β and MIP-1α among unstimulated mouse epidermal cells, *Journal of Investigative Dermatology*, **99**, 537–41.

METLAY, J.P., PURE, E. and STEINMAN, R.M., 1989, Control of the immune response at the level of antigen presenting cells: a comparison of the function of dendritic cells and B lymphocytes, *Advances in Immunology*, **47**, 45–116.

MILLER, A.E. and LEVIS, W.R., 1973, Studies on the contact sensitization of man with simple chemicals. I. Specific lymphocyte transformation in response to dinitrochlorobenzene sensitization, *Journal of Investigative Dermatology*, **61**, 261–9.

MOULON, C., PEGUET-NAVARRO, J., COURTELLEMONT, P., REDZINIAK, G. and SCHMITT, D., 1993, In vitro primary sensitization and restimulation of hapten-specific T cells by fresh and cultured human epidermal Langerhans cells, *Immunology*, **80**, 373–9.

MOULON, C., PEGUET-NAVARRO, J., COURTELLEMONT, P., REDZINIAK, G. and SCHMITT, D., 1994, Hapten presentation by human epidermal Langerhans cells in vitro, in Rougier, A., Goldberg, A.M. and Maibach, H.I. (eds), *In Vitro Skin Toxicology, Irritation, Phototoxicity, Sensitization*, pp. 313–23, New York: Mary Ann Liebert.

NICOLAS, J-F., GARRIGUE, J-L., BOUR, H. and SCHMITT, D., 1994, Secondary T cell response to haptens in vitro: a step towards an entirely in vitro screening assay for contact sensitizers, in Rougier, A., Goldberg, A.M. and Maibach, H.I. (eds), *In Vitro Skin Toxicology, Irritation, Phototoxicity, Sensitization*, pp. 333–40, New York: Mary Ann Liebert.

PASTORE, S., SHIVJI, G.M., KONDO, S., KONO, T., McKENZIE, R.C., SEGAL, L., SOMERS, D. and SAUDER, D.N., 1995, Effects of contact sensitizers neomycin sulfate, benzocaine and 2,4-dinitrobenzene 1-sulfonate sodium salt on viability, membrane integrity and IL-1α mRNA expression of cultured normal human keratinocytes, *Toxicology in Vitro*, **33**, 57–68.

PHANUPHAK, P., MOORHEAD, J.W. and CLAMAN, H.N., 1974, Tolerance and contact sensitivity to DNFB in mice. II. Specific in vitro stimulation with a hapten, 2,4-dinitrobenzene sulfonic acid (DNBSO$_3$,Na), *Journal of Immunology*, **112**, 549–51.

PICUT, C.A., LEE, C.S. and LEWIS, R.M., 1987, Ultrastructural and phenotypic change in Langerhans cells induced in vitro by contact allergens, *British Journal of Dermatology*, **116**, 773–84.

ROBINSON, M.K., 1989, Optimization of an in vitro lymphocyte blastogenesis assay for predictive assessment of immunologic responsiveness to contact sensitizers, *Journal of Investigative Dermatology*, **92**, 860–7.

ROBINSON, M.K. and SNELLER, D.L., 1990, Use of an optimized in vitro lymphocyte blastogenesis assay to detect contact sensitivity to nickel sulfate in mice, *Toxicology and Applied Pharmacology*, **104**, 106–16.

SANTIAGO-SCHWARZ, F., BELILOS, E., DIAMOND, B. and CARSONS, S.E., 1992, TNF in combination with GM-CSF enhances the differentiation of neonatal cord blood stem cells into dendritic cells and macrophages, *Journal of Leukocyte Biology*, **52**, 274–81.

SARLO, K. and CLARK, E.D., 1992, A tier approach for evaluating the respiratory allergenicity of low molecular weight chemicals, *Fundamental and Applied Toxicology*, **18**, 107–14.

SCHREIBER, S., KILGUS, O., PAYER, E., KUTIL, R. ELBE, A., MUELLER, C. and STINGL, G., 1992, Cytokine pattern of Langerhans cells isolated from murine epidermal cell cultures, *Journal of Immunology*, **149**, 3525–34.

SCHULER, G. and STEINMAN, R.M., 1985, Murine epidermal Langerhans cells mature into potent immunostimulatory dendritic cells in vitro, *Journal of Experimental Medicine*, **161**, 526–46.

SOEBERG, B. and ANDERSON, V., 1976, Hapten-specific lymphocyte transformation in humans sensitized with NDMA or DNCB, *Clinical and Experimental Immunology*, **25**, 490–2.

TREDE, N.S., GEHA, R.S. and CHATILA, T., 1991, Transcriptional activation of IL-1β and tumor necrosis factor-α genes by MHC class II ligands, *Journal of Immunology*, **146**, 2310–5.

VON BLOMBERG-VAN DER FLIER, B.M.E., BRUYNZEEL, D.P. and SCHEPER, R.J., 1989, Impact of 25 years of in vitro testing in allergic contact dermatitis, in Frosch, P.J., Dooms-Goossens, A., Lachapelle, J-M., Rycroft, R.J.G. and Scheper, R.J. (eds), *Current Topics in Contact Dermatitis*, pp. 569–77, Heidelberg: Springer-Verlag.

VON BLOMBERG-VAN DER FLIER, M., VAN DER BURG, C.K.H., POS, O., VAN DE PLASSCHE-BOERS, E.M., BRUYNZEEL, D.P., GAROTTA, G. and SCHEPER, R.J., 1987, In vitro studies in nickel allergy: diagnostic value of dual parameter analysis. *Journal of Investigative Dermatology*, **88**, 362–8.

WILMER, J.L., BURLESON, F.G., KAYAMA, F., KANNO, J. and LUSTER, M.I., 1994, Cytokine induction in human epidermal keratinocytes exposed to contact irritants and its relation to chemical-induced inflammation in mouse skin, *Journal of Investigative Dermatology*, **102**, 915–22.

YAMADA, M., NIWA, Y., FUJIMOTO, F. and YOSHINAGA, H., 1972, Lymphocyte transformation in allergic contact dermatitis, *Japanese Journal of Dermatology*, **82**, 94–7.

151

10

Risk Assessment

D.A. BASKETTER

Unilever Environmental Safety Laboratory, Sharnbrook

G.F. GERBERICK and M.K. ROBINSON

Procter and Gamble, Cincinnati

Introduction

Allergic contact dermatitis (ACD) is a relatively common disorder in man, particularly in an occupational setting (Coenraads and Smit, 1995). It is instructive to consider why this is the case. Clinical ACD requires that humans be exposed sufficiently to contact allergens in the absence of appropriate risk management procedures, in other words, where there is a combination of a contact allergenic hazard with inadequately controlled exposure. However, it is evident from a wealth of published literature (e.g. Wahlberg and Boman, 1985; Botham *et al.*, 1991a; Cronin and Basketter, 1994; Kimber *et al.*, 1994, together with Chapters 7 and 8 in this present volume) that adequate methods have existed for some time which enable toxicologists to identify chemicals that present a contact allergenic hazard. Thus it is reasonable to speculate that the current prevalence of ACD arises, at least in part, from a continuing failure adequately to understand and/or implement risk assessment/management procedures when there is a reasonable possibility of skin exposure to potential contact allergens. In this chapter, it is our aim to provide detailed guidance on the processes of risk assessment that should be applied in such cases. Risk assessment is of fundamental importance – skin sensitization tests in general only evaluate hazards, and to some extent their potency. The risk assessment process enables these abstract hazards to be placed in a practical context and, where appropriate, permit risk management measures to be defined. Manufacturers of consumer and health care products, that come into direct contact with the skin, have a major responsibility to the consumer and to the worker to ensure that products will not cause allergic contact dermatitis. Product and ingredient safety assessment should consider all types of human exposure situations. This includes the manufacture and distribution of the product as well as consumer use and reasonably foreseeable misuse. The guidance presented herein is based on our many years of experience of making risk assessments for large companies which manufacture a wide range of products which come into contact with the skin of billions of consumers.

It is critical to understand that, in spite of the decision-tree approach often used to illustrate the testing and risk assessment process (Gerberick *et al.*, 1993), the process itself is neither static nor prescriptive. Each step in such approaches requires the toxicologist carefully to evaluate available data on the chemical or formulation relative to benchmark materials and the type of exposure expected in the workplace and the home. Furthermore, it should be noted that the clinical testing discussed below is flexible to permit evaluation of the chemical or formulation that may be unique to the product type and allow easier prediction of sensitization risk to workers or consumers. For example, there may be one testing format that is most appropriate for a liquid laundry detergent, with limited or transient exposure to hands, and another for a liquid dishwashing detergent with more chronic exposure under high-temperature hand-immersion conditions. On the other hand, the risk assessment for a transdermal drug, which includes an element of health benefit, is different from an antiperspirant which carries only a cosmetic benefit. Examples of the testing and risk assessment process from benchmark laundry detergent additives have been extensively reviewed previously (Robinson *et al.*, 1989; Calvin, 1992).

Preliminary Considerations

The basic process to be employed for evaluating the skin sensitization risk is essentially a comparative toxicological approach. It is the potential for an adverse effect to occur in humans exposed during manufacturing or product use that is being determined. This approach incorporates the assessment of both toxicity and exposure of the new ingredient followed by a comparison of these data with the toxicity and exposure data for known safe and potentially unsafe chemicals and product formulations. In assessing skin sensitization risk, the level of exposure to the material as well as the material's inherent toxicity needs to be determined. The key factors considered in exposure assessment for skin sensitization include chemical dose, chemical biovailability, concentration in dose/unit surface area (Upadhye and Maibach, 1992), duration of exposure, body location, presence of any skin penetration aid or vehicle, primary skin irritation potential, and the extent of occlusion of the exposed skin. Relevant to determining conditions of exposure for consumer use of products is the gathering of habits and practices data for each chemical or product type. These data include the frequency and duration of each product use activity and the dose of product inherent to that particular habit or practice. All exposure information is incorporated into the planning of and evaluation of the results from predictive skin sensitization tests.

However, before embarking on a detailed/documented risk assessment, it is important to consider a few simple points. Firstly, risk assessment is not a highly prescriptive process that should always be followed in the same way. On the contrary, what is necessary is that it is carried out thoroughly to the point where the risk has been adequately assessed. In some circumstances, this point may be reached quite quickly and with minimal expenditure of time and effort. In other cases, substantial and sustained effort is required. For example, in what is an admittedly relatively obvious situation, when exposure to the contact allergen is essentially zero, then even for highly potent contact allergens, there is no need to go further with a risk assessment. ACD will not occur. Furthermore, if the exposure is sufficiently low, then it may not be necessary to know precisely the potency of a contact allergen. Simply the knowledge that it is not a very strong allergen may be sufficient to permit a proper conclusion of the risk assessment. Another situation where risk assessment may be relatively simple is the replacement of an ingredient with another of the same or similar type (e.g. an alternative supplier of a raw material). In such a case, and where the risk is already known to be very low, all that may be necessary is to confirm that the specification of the new source of raw material is the same. Alternatively, data which provide evidence that the relative sensitization potential of the old and new materials is similar may suffice. In contrast, even where the intrinsic sensitization potential is very low, if skin contact is sufficiently intense and prolonged, then sensitization may occur. An example of this is the situation where medicaments are applied continuously to skin, often damaged and/or inflamed skin, under occlusion. A prime example is found with stasis ulcers, where a variety of medicaments and chemicals with negligible sensitization potential, such as cetostearyl alcohol and paraben esters, quite frequently cause ACD.

Analytical Characterization and Literature Review

When a more detailed risk assessment is required, this may involve review of analytical data on the material and review of the published literature for any evidence suggestive of skin sensitization potential. Obviously, if adequate published literature on the sensitization potential of the material of interest is available, further testing may not be required. Appropriate analytical information may come from the supplier or from the product development group. Important in the risk assessment process is the identification of materials that may raise issues regarding sensitization potential based on their physical and chemical properties (e.g. low molecular weight with functional groups that may interact with cell surface proteins) (Dupuis and Benezra,

1982; Barratt *et al.*, 1994; Basketter *et al.*, 1995). In addition, any expected contaminants or reaction by-products with known sensitization properties need to be evaluated. If any such materials are identified, analytical work can be conducted to have the allergic contaminants removed or controlled to safe, non-sensitizing levels (Lindup and Nowell, 1977; Roberts *et al.*, 1990).

Animal Test Methods in the Risk Assessment Process

Skin sensitization testing can provide essential safety data on new ingredients or formulations which lack adequate sensitization data. Whilst very many protocols are available, the skin sensitization tests most commonly used are the guinea pig maximization test (GPMT) (Magnusson and Kligman, 1970), the Buehler occluded patch test (Robinson *et al.*, 1990) and the murine local lymph node assay (Gerberick *et al.*, 1992, see Chapters 7 and 8).

The GPMT and Buehler methods have been used by us for over 20 years for assessing inherent contact sensitization potential of materials prior to human exposure. When properly conducted and interpreted, these tests have demonstrated the ability to detect chemicals with moderate to strong sensitization potential as well as those with relatively weak sensitization potential (Robinson *et al.*, 1990; Botham *et al.*, 1991a; Basketter and Scholes, 1992). In addition to using these tests to assess inherent contact sensitization potential, they have also been useful in addressing question of sensitization potency of antigenic cross-reactivity of structurally similar chemicals, identification of chemical contaminants in raw materials, or comparison of the sensitization potential of a raw material produced by different chemical processes (e.g. Ritz *et al.*, 1975; Basketter and Goodwin, 1989; Botham *et al.*, 1991a).

Data from such methods can be used in the development of a comparative risk assessment. In principle, results with an unknown material can be evaluated in the context of the database of results of known contact allergens and non-allergens. Such an approach can be adopted only where the sensitivity and consistency of the sensitization method at the testing institution are well known and properly understood. The data must of course be interpreted in the context of the test concentrations, vehicles and the incidence and intensity of any sensitization reactions. Where a chemical is likely to have extensive skin contact at a significant concentration, only the most sensitive of test methods can be expected to provide an adequate assessment of intrinsic sensitization potential. It should be noted that this does not mean that materials which cause skin sensitization cannot be used safely, i.e. with very low risk of causing allergic contact dermatitis. Even for the most potent contact allergens there is a safe dose. The task before the risk assessor is to determine the exposure conditions commensurate with this safe dose.

The major guinea pig skin sensitization test methods used to test the sensitization potential of new materials have a solid track record to date. The adjuvant methods, particularly the GPMT, are generally considered most sensitive in terms of sensitization hazard identification (Andersen and Maibach, 1985), although comparison of results with occluded patch testing, at least on selected materials, often indicates comparable results (Robinson *et al.*, 1989). Indeed the patch test methods may be more readily extrapolated in the context of risk assessment. Examples of known clinical skin sensitizers identifiable by occluded patch testing of guinea pigs but formulated at generally safe levels into consumer products and medicaments include Kathon CG, benzoyl peroxide, hydroxycitronellal and cinnamic aldehyde (Steltenkamp *et al.*, 1980; Chan *et al.*, 1983; Buehler, 1985; Danneman *et al.*, 1983).

Recently, Kimber and others have developed and proposed the use of a mouse local lymph node assay (LLNA) for use in screening materials for their contact sensitization potential (Kimber *et al.*, 1986; Kimber and Weisenberger, 1989; Kimber *et al.*, 1989). The LLNA measures the induction phase of contact sensitization by determining the ability of a chemical to stimulate the incorporation of radiolabelled thymidine into proliferating lymph node cells in a small number of animals. The LLNA offers the advantages of 1) requiring less time for completion, 2) an objective endpoint, 3) requiring approximately half the number of animals compared with traditional guinea pig methods, and 4) being less costly than most currently employed guinea pig test methods. Results of validation studies (Kimber and Weisenberger, 1989; Kimber *et al.*, 1989; Gerberick *et al.*, 1992) indicate that the assay is able to detect strong, moderate and some weak sensitizers. Moreover, interlaboratory comparisons have demonstrated that the LLNA is a robust and reliable method for the identification of moderate and strong contact allergens and demonstrates good concordance with guinea pig test data (Kimber *et al.*, 1990, 1991, 1994; Basketter *et al.*, 1991; Basketter and Scholes, 1992). Based on these results, we believe the assay is a useful test to incorporate into a scheme for contact sensitization risk assessment (Gerberick *et al.*, 1992). Botham *et al.* (1991b) and Basketter *et al.* (1992) have demonstrated that the LLNA is more amenable than other animal sensitization tests for the assessment of relative potency.

Human Test Methods in the Risk Assessment Process

Human Maximization Test

This test was described in detail by Kligman (1966) as a rigorous and sensitive predictive assay for the identification of the sensitization potential of chemicals. Further commentary was made on the technique some 9 years later (Kligman and Epstein, 1975). In principle, a group of 25 subjects is subjected

156

to repeated 48-hour occlusive patch treatment with as high a concentration of test chemical as possible on five occasions over a two week period. If the substance is not sufficiently irritating, the irritancy is enhanced by prior treatment of the site for 24-hours with sodium lauryl sulphate prior to each 48-hour patch. The extent of sensitization in the panel is assessed by 48-hour occluded patch challenge one week after completion of the five induction treatments on a slightly irritated skin site using the maximum non-irritant concentration of the test substance. The challenge sites are scored at 48-hours and 96-hours post-application. The original publication (Kligman, 1966) which reports details of test results on about 90 chemicals of widely varying sensitization potential amply demonstrates the sensitivity of the protocol. In essence, this procedure can provide a stringent assessment of intrinsic sensitization hazard and its relative potency. However, its practical application is limited by ethical considerations.

Human Repeat Insult Patch Test (HRIPT)

Alternatively, the HRIPT can be carried out, usually in a manner designed to provide a more direct evaluation of risk or lack thereof. Generally, 80–120 test subjects are employed (Stotts, 1980). The induction phase of the HRIPT includes nine 24-hour patches at a single site with a 24-hour rest between patches (48-hours on weekends). The concentration of material tested is determined by integrating the following factors: prior sensitization test results, the assessment of skin irritation in repeated application patch studies in humans, the desire to exaggerate the exposure relative to anticipated normal use/misuse exposure (if irritancy considerations permit), and prior experience. It is often preferred that a material be tested at the highest minimally irritating concentration as determined in a human irritation screen. After induction, there is then a 14–17 day rest, followed by a 24-hour challenge patch applied on the original and a naive skin site. In general, skin reactions are scored during induction (just prior to patch reapplication), and 24- and 72-hours after challenge patch removal, although scores from 48-hours, 96-hours, and even longer intervals after challenge may be included. Contact sensitization reactions are generally characterized by erythema along with various dermal sequelae (e.g., edema, papules, vesicles, and bullae). A characteristic sensitization response that occurs and persists during challenge at both the original and alternate (naive) patch sites is considered indicative of sensitization and should be confirmed by appropriate re-challenge. The challenge of both the original and naive sites, the delayed scoring, and the re-challenge procedure maximize the sensitivity and reliability of the test procedure.

The HRIPT can provide an exaggeration of anticipated product use/misuse exposures through an extended duration of exposure, testing higher than use concentrations, minor skin irritation of the test material, and, for many

157

product types, through the occluded patch. The procedure allows the detection of pre-existing sensitization to the test material (chemical or final formulation) as confirmed by persistent skin reactions early in the induction period. Any positive or questionable response during the induction phase or only during the challenge phase is investigated further by a re-challenge patch study. Here a dose-response study may be conducted to determine whether a response elicitation threshold can be established. In addition, sensitizers in formulations can be identified via re-challenge. It is important to note, however, that the HRIPT is not done to predict or to identify sensitization potential but to confirm safety under exaggerated conditions relative to anticipated consumer exposure.

In addition to the important preclinical data generated, confirmation that humans will not adversely respond provides additional and sometimes essential data for safety programmes designed to assess the skin sensitization risk of new chemicals and products. The data generated in HRIPT are combined with data from the mouse and/or guinea pig, and worker and consumer exposure and compared with the data on relevant benchmark materials to give a revised assessment of risk. Depending on the sensitization data generated, the exposure calculations and comparison with benchmarks, a decision may be reached to either stop development (Robinson *et al.*, 1991) or to obtain additional clinical data in carefully controlled use tests under more realistic exposure conditions before proceeding with a new chemical ingredient for product development (e.g. Calvin, 1992).

Provocative Use Testing of Sensitized Subjects

Individuals showing patch test sensitization reactions to a material may be asked to participate in extended provocative use testing of a product containing the putative sensitizing agent. The individual(s) may have been sensitized by HRIPT, identified as pre-sensitized during the course of the HRIPT or identified by diagnostic patch test screening. Because of the relative rarity of sensitization in available study populations, the numbers of individuals in provocative use tests usually are small. However, test group size is not the critical factor, since the question being asked is whether elicitation of allergic contact dermatitis will occur when the test product is used by someone known to be sensitized to the formula or ingredient under patch test conditions. A provocative use test is considered to be of minimal risk as long as there is sufficient exaggeration inherent in the HRIPT or exposure is highly localized. However, before conducting any use test, a formal risk assessment is done to verify there is minimal risk of eliciting allergic reactions. The risk assessment should include an evaluation of patch test versus in use exposure concentrations, frequency of exposure, a comparison with results obtained previously on benchmark formulations, and, if necessary, the results of an open application test. At the conclusion of the use test, even if no adverse skin effects were observed, a follow-up diagnostic patch test should be done to confirm that the test subject is still reactive under patch test conditions.

In some instances, individuals reactive to ingredients under exaggerated patch test exposure conditions do not react when exposed to the ingredient in the context of normal product use (Nusair *et al.*, 1988; Robinson *et al.*, 1989). An illustrative example is provided by the chemical preservative Kathon CG. Occluded patch sensitization testing in guinea pigs indicated that concentrations as low as 25 parts per million (ppm) could induce sensitization (Chan *et al.*, 1983). Subsequent human repeat insult patch testing identified the sensitization threshold (under patch) in man as 12.5–20 ppm (Cardin *et al.*, 1986). Pre-sensitized subjects could safely use various 'rinse off' products (e.g. shampoo, hair conditioner, fabric softener, bath or shower foam) formulated with 4–6 ppm of Kathon CG (Weaver *et al.*, 1985). Nevertheless, higher concentrations in 'leave on' products have been associated with a significant incidence of allergic contact dermatitis (de Groot and Weyland, 1988; de Groot, 1990), emphasizing the importance of making a careful risk assessment. In contrast, in the case of a transdermal antihistamine product, positive skin reactions under open application test conditions confirmed both the nature (allergic contact sensitization) and relevance of the skin reactions to the active drug providing compelling evidence to support discontinuation of the project (Robinson *et al.*, 1991).

Extended Use Testing

The extended prospective use test is a method used to determine the potential for a product to induce sensitization or both induce sensitization and elicit allergic skin reactions under typical conditions of product use. As in the other clinical studies, a formal risk assessment is done, written fully informed consent is obtained and expert dermatologist monitoring and assessment of any skin reactions is included in the protocol. The number of test subjects and the length of a prospective use test is dependent on the product being evaluated. Generally, prospective use tests can include 100 to 500 subjects and extend three to six months. Diagnostic patch testing at the conclusion of the study can be done to verify lack of patch test reactivity or to identify subclinical sensitization responses (i.e. subjects with induced sensitization but no clinical dermatitis). Any evidence of induced sensitization would necessitate consideration of withholding a developmental product or ingredient from the market.

One indication of the dynamic nature of the testing and risk assessment process is illustrated by the example of a programme to develop olefin sulphonates (AOS) for liquid dishwashing detergents (Robinson *et al.*, 1989). Extensive initial testing of AOS and formulation containing AOS (guinea pig skin sensitization tests, HRIPT, and diagnostic testing of the general population) had shown slight but potentially acceptable sensitization risk from the dishwashing formula. However, due to the extreme exposure conditions (hot water, hand immersion, surfactant matrix) and presence of low levels of unsaturated sultones (potent skin sensitizers, Ritz *et al.*, 1975) in the AOS, the decision was made to run a prospective use test in volunteers. In this study, two subjects (without pre-sensitization to AOS or sultone) out of 264 using AOS-containing product at home developed skin reactions. These reactions were confirmed in controlled re-use testing, and proven to be due to AOS by diagnostic patch testing. It was through this flexible testing approach, initiated because of the chemical in question (the presence of strongly sensitizing sultone contaminants) and nature of product use, that the consumer risk was firmly established and this AOS-containing product application discontinued (Robinson *et al.*, 1989). Modern manufacturing procedures which essentially eliminate the unacceptable sultone contaminant may thus provide the only route to safe use of AOS in this situation (de Groot, 1994).

Prior to marketing, all preclinical and clinical data are incorporated into a formal risk assessment for the chemical and product formulation in question. In the risk assessment, the data should again be compared with appropriate benchmarks. In some instances it is appropriate to obtain outside expert opinion and concurrence for any new ingredient that shows evidence of inducing skin sensitization in humans, even if only under exaggerated conditions of skin exposure.

Monitoring and Follow-Up of Consumer Comments

Contact sensitization risk assessment does not end with the decision to manufacture/market the product. All comments related to skin safety that are received from the exposed population can be collated, evaluated and, if appropriate, investigated by medical personnel. In some instances, follow-up may involve diagnostic patch testing of the product and/or selected product ingredients to determine the relationship, if any, between the product in question and the skin reaction. Another method that can be used to obtain skin sensitization data among consumers is to conduct diagnostic patch test surveys and to distribute questionnaires about skin effects among consumers who have used the product. Control subjects (non-users) of approximately equal age, gender, and other comparable factors, as well as control test substances and products, should be included in these studies. The data are useful not only in confirming the validity of the risk assessment, but also in detecting potential problems. Post-market monitoring provides both the ongoing assurance of product safety as well as additional benchmark data for comparison with other ingredient and product initiatives that follow.

Conclusion

This review describes an approach that has been used to assess the skin sensitization risk, particularly in relation to new product ingredients prior to and after marketing and which we consider encapsulates the essential elements which need to be applied to any risk assessment for skin sensitization. In particular, the risk assessment process utilizes a comparative toxicological approach in which data on the inherent sensitization potential of a material and the exposure to it through manufacturing or consumer use or foreseeable misuse are integrated and compared with data generated by 'benchmark' materials, usually of similar chemistry or product application, or both. This approach has proven itself by providing an accurate assessment of skin sensitization potential and the basis for eventual safe marketing of a wide range of consumer household and personal care products and topical pharmaceuticals. By the use of thorough but not prescriptive risk assessment processes, and the coupling of these with appropriate risk management practices, it is possible to minimize the occurrence of ACD.

References

ANDERSEN, K.E. and MAIBACH, H.I., 1985, Guinea pig sensitization assays: An overview, in Andersen, K.E. and Maibach, H.I. (eds), *Contact Allergy Predictive Tests in Guinea Pigs, Current Problems in Dermatology*, Vol. 14, pp. 59–106, New York: Karger.

BARRATT, M.D., BASKETTER, D.A., CHAMBERLAIN, M., ADMANS, G. and LANGOWSKI, J., 1994, An expert system rulebase for identifying contact allergens. *Toxicology in Vitro*, **8**, 1053–60.

BASKETTER, D.A., DOOMS-GOOSSENS, A., KALBERG, A-T. and LEPOITTEVIN, J-P., 1995, The chemistry of contact allergy: why is a molecule allergenic?, *Contact Dermatitis*, **32**, 65–73.

BASKETTER, D.A. and GOODWIN, B.F.J. 1989, Investigation of the prohapten concept. Cross reactions between 1,4-substituted benzene derivatives in the guinea pig. *Contact Dermatitis*, **19**, 248–53.

BASKETTER, D.A., ROBERTS, D.W., CRONIN, M. and SCHOLES, E.W., 1992, The value of the local lymph node assay in quantitative structure activity investigations. *Contact Dermatitis*, **27**, 137–42.

BASKETTER, D.A. and SCHOLES, E.W., 1992, A comparison of the local lymph node assay with the guinea pig maximisation test for the detection of a range of contact allergens. *Food and Chemical Toxicology*, **30**, 65–9.

BASKETTER, D.A., SCHOLES, E.W., KIMBER, I., BOTHAM, P.A., HILTON, J., MILLER, K., ROBBINS, M.C., HARRISON, P.T.C. and WAITE, S.J., 1991, Interlaboratory evaluation of the local lymph node assay with 25 chemicals and comparison with guinea pig test data. *Toxicology Methods*, **1**, 30–43.

BOTHAM, P.A., BASKETTER, D.A., MAURER, TH., MUELLER, D., POTOKAR, M. and BONTINCK, W.J., 1991a, Skin sensitization – a critical review of predictive test methods in animal and man. *Food and Chemical Toxicology*, **29**, 275–86.

BOTHAM, P.A., HILTON, J., EVANS, C.D., LEES, D. and HALL, T.J., 1991b, Assessment of the relative skin sensitizing potency of 3 biocides using the murine local lymph node assay. *Contact Dermatitis*, **25**, 172–7.

BUEHLER, E.V., 1985, A rationale for the selection of occlusion to induce and elicit delayed contact hypersensivity in the guinea pig, in Andersen, K.E. and Maibach, H.I. (eds.), *Current Problems in Dermatology*, Vol. 14, pp. 39–58, New York: Karger.

CALVIN, G., 1992, Risk management case history – detergents, in Richardson, M.L. (ed.), *Risk Management of Chemicals*, pp. 120–36, London: Royal Society of Chemistry.

CARDIN, C.W., WEAVER, J.E. and BAILEY, P.T., 1986, Dose response assessments of Kathon biocide. (II) Threshold prophetic patch testing, *Contact Dermatitis*, **15**, 10–16.

CHAN, P.D., BALDWIN, R.C., PARSON, R.D., MOSS, J.N., STEROTELLI, R., SMITH, J.M. and HAYES, A.W., 1983, Kathon biocide: manifestation of delayed contact dermatitis in guinea pigs is dependent on the concentration for induction and challenge. *Journal of Investigative Dermatology*, **81**, 409–11.

COENRAADS, P-J. and SMIT, J., 1995, Epidemiology, in Rycroft, R.J.G., Frosch, P., Benezra, C. and Menne, T. (eds.), *Textbook of Contact Dermatitis*, 2nd edn, Heidelberg: Springer Verlag.

CRONIN, M.T.D. and BASKETTER, D.A., 1994, Multivariate QSAR analysis of a skin sensitization database. *SAR and QSAR in Environmental Research*, **2**, 159–79.

DANNEMAN, P.J., BOOMAN, K.A., DORSKY, J., KOHRMAN, K.A., ROTHENSTEIN, A.S., SEDLAK, R.I., STELTENKAMP, R.J. and THOMPSON, G.R., 1983, Cinnamic aldehyde: a survey of consumer patch test sensitization. *Food and Chemical Toxicology*, **21**, 721–5.

DE GROOT, A.C., 1990, Methylisothiazolinone/methylchloroisothiazolinone (Kathon CG) allergy: an updated review. *American Journal of Contact Dermatitis*, **1**, 151–6.

DE GROOT, A.C. and WEYLAND, J.W., 1988, Kathon, C.G.: a review. *Journal of the American Academy of Dermatology*, **18**, 350–8.

DE GROOT, W.H., 1994, *Sulphonation Technology in the Detergent Industry*. Dordrecht: Kluwer.

DUPUIS, G. and BENEZRA, C., 1982, *Allergic Contact Dermatitis to Simple Chemicals. A Molecular Approach*, New York: Marcel Dekker.

GERBERICK, G.F., HOUSE, R.V., FLETCHER, E.R. and RYAN, C.A., 1992, Examination of the local lymph mode assay for use in contact sensitization risk assessment. *Fundamental and Applied Toxicology*, **19**, 438–45.

GERBERICK, G.F., ROBINSON, M.K. and STOTTS, J., 1993, An approach to allergic contact sensitization risk assessment of new chemicals and product ingredients. *American Journal of Contact Dermatitis*, **4**, 205–11.

KIMBER, I., DEARMAN, R.J., SCHOLES, E.W. and BASKETTER, D.A., 1994, The local lymph node assay: developments and applications. *Toxicology*, **93**, 13–31.

KIMBER, I., HILTON, J. and BOTHAM, P.A., 1990, Identification of contact allergens using the murine local lymph node assay: comparisons with the Buehler occluded patch test in guinea pigs. *Journal of Applied Toxicology*, **10**, 173–80.

KIMBER, I., HILTON, J., BOTHAM, P.A., BASKETTER, D.A. and SCHOLES, E.W., MILLER, K., ROBBINS, M.C., HARRISON, P.T.C., GRAY, T.J.B. and WAITE, S.J., 1991, The murine local lymph node assay: results of an inter-laboratory trial. *Toxicology Letters*, **55**, 203–13.

KIMBER, I., HILTON, J. and WEISENBERGER, C., 1989, The murine local lymph node assay for identification of contact allergens: a preliminary evaluation of in situ measurement of lymphocyte proliferation. *Contact Dermatitis*, **21**, 215–20.

KIMBER, I., MITCHELL, J.A. and GRIFFIN, A.C., 1986, Development of a murine local lymph node assay for the determination of sensitizing potential. *Food and Chemical Toxicology*, **24**, 585–6.

KIMBER, I. and WEISENBERGER, C., 1989, A murine local lymph node assay for the identification of contact allergens. Assay development and results of an inttial validation study. *Archives of Toxicolǫgy*, **63**, 274–82.

KLIGMAN, A.M., 1966, The identification of contact allergens by human assay. III, *Journal of Investigative Dermatology*, **47**, 393–409.

KLIGMAN, A.M. and EPSTEIN, W., 1975, Updating the maximization test for identifying contact allergens. *Contact Dermatitis*, **1**, 231–9.

LINDUP, W.E. and NOWELL, P.T., 1977, Role of sultone contaminants in an outbreak of allergic contact dermatitis caused by alkyl ethoxysulphates: a review. *Food and Cosmetic Toxicology*, **16**, 59–62.

MAGNUSSON, B. and KLIGMAN, A.M., 1970, *Allergic Contact Dermatitis in the Guinea Pig*, Philadelphia: Charles C. Thomas.

NUSAIR, T.L., DANNEMAN, P.J., STOTTS, J. and BAY, P.H.S., 1988, Consumer products: risk assessment process for contact sensitization. *Toxicologist*, **8**, 258–64.

RITZ, H.L., CONNOR, D.S. and SAUTER, E.D., 1975, Contact sensitization of guinea-pigs with unsaturated and halogenated sultones. *Contact Dermatitis*, **1**, 349–51.

ROBERTS, D.W., LAWRENCE, J.G., FAIRWEATHER, I.A., CLEMETT, C.J. and SAUL, C.D., 1990, Alk-1-ene-1,3-sultones in a-olefin sulphonates. *Tenside Surfactants and Detergents*, **27**, 82–6.

ROBINSON, M.K., PARSELL, K.W., BRENEMAN, D.L. and CRUZE, C.A., 1991, Evaluation of the primary skin sensitization and allergic contact sensitization potential of transdermal triprolidone. *Fundamental and Applied Toxicology*, **17**, 103–19.

ROBINSON, M.K., NUSAIR, T.L., FLETCHER, E.R. and RITZ, H.L., 1990, A review of the Buehler guinea pig skin sensitization test and its use in a risk assessment process for human skin sensitization. *Toxicology*, **61**, 91–107.

ROBINSON, M.K., STOTTS, J., DANNEMAN, P.J., NUSAIR, T.L. and BAY, P.H.S., 1989, A risk assessment process for allergic contact sensitization. *Food and Chemical Toxicology*, **27**, 479–89.

STELTENKAMP, R.J., BOOMAN, K.A., DORSKY, J., KING, T.O., ROTHENSTEIN, A.S., SCHWOEPPE, E.A., SEDLAK, R.I., SMITH, T.H. and THOMPSON, G.R., 1980, Hydroxycitronellal: a survey of consumer patch test sensitization. *Food and Chemical Toxicology*, **18**, 407–12.

STOTTS, J., 1980, Planning, conduct, and interpretation of human predictive sensitization patch tests, in *Current Concepts in Cutaneous Toxicity*, V.A. Drill and P. Lazer (eds), pp. 41–55, Academic Press: New York,

UPADHYE, M.R. and MAIBACH, H.I., 1992, Influence of area of application of allergen on sensitization in contact dermatitis. *Contact Dermatitis*, **27**, 281–6.

WAHLBERG, J.E. and BOMAN, A., 1985, Guinea pig maximisation test, in Andersen, K.E. and Maibach, H.I. (eds), *Current Problems in Dermatology*, Vol. 14, pp. 59–106, New York: Karger.

WEAVER, J.E., CARDIN, C.W. and MAIBACH, H.I., 1985, Dose response assessments of Kathon biocide. I. Diagnostic use and diagnostic threshold patch testing with sensitized humans. *Contact Dermatitis*, **12**, 141–5.

Index

165